20·99

Manual Therapy Masterclasses

The Peripheral Joints

For Churchill Livingstone:

Commissioning Editor: Mary Law
Development Editor: Kim Benson
Project Manager: Lucy Thorburn
Production Manager: Marina Maher
Layout: Spot on Creative
Cover Design: Marie Prime

Manual Therapy Masterclasses
The Peripheral Joints

Edited by

Karen S. Beeton

Principal Lecturer, Department of Allied Health Professions — Physiotherapy
University of Hertfordshire, Hatfield, United Kingdom

Foreword by

Ann P Moore and **Gwendolen A Jull**

CHURCHILL LIVINGSTONE

EDINBURGH LONDON NEW YORK OXFORD PHILADELPHIA ST LOUIS SYDNEY TORONTO 2003

Churchill Livingstone
An imprint of Elsevier Limited.

ISBN 0 443 07402 X

British Library Cataloguing in Publication Data
A catalogue record for this book is available from the British
Library.

Library of Congress Cataloging in Publication Data
A catalog record for this book is available from the Library of
Congress.

Note
Medical knowledge is constantly changing. As new
information becomes available, changes in treatment,
procedures, equipment and the use of drugs become
necessary. The author/contributors and the publishers have
taken great care to ensure that the information given in this
text is accurate and up to date. However, readers are strongly
advised to confirm that the information, especially with
regard to drug usage, complies with the latest legislation and
standards of practice.

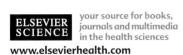

your source for books,
journals and multimedia
in the health sciences
www.elsevierhealth.com

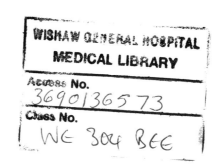
The
Publisher's
policy is to use
**paper manufactured
from sustainable forests**

Printed by Grafos S.A. Arte sobre papel, Spain.

Contents

Contributors

Jill L. Cook
Senior Lecturer, Musculoskeletal Research Centre, La Trobe University, Bundoora, Victoria, Australia

Fiona J. Coutts
Principal Lecturer, Department of Physiotherapy School of Health Science, University of East London, London, United Kingdom

Linda Exelby
Clinical Specialist, Pinehill Hospital, Hitchin, North Herts, United Kingdom

Sally A. Hess
Department of Physiotherapy, The University of Queensland, St. Lucia, Brisbane, Queensland, Australia

Glenn Hunter
Department of Physiotherapy and Occupational Therapy, University of the West of England, Bristol, United Kingdom

Karim Khan
Sports Physician, Department of Family Practice and Orthopaedics, University of British Columbia, Vancouver, BC, Canada

Linda M.G. Lang
Sheffield Hallam University, School of Health & Social Care, Collegiate Campus, Sheffield, United Kingdom

Dana J. Lawrence
Postgraduate Dean and Director, Department of Editorial Review and Publication, National University of Health Sciences, Lombard, Illinois, USA

Jenny McConnell
McConnell and Clements Physiotherapy, Mosman, Sydney, New South Wales, Australia

Sarah L. Mottram
Director, Kinetic Control, Southampton, United Kingdom

Craig Purdam
Head of Physiotherapy and Massage, Australian Institute of Sport, Canberra, Australia

Kevin J. Sims
Department of Physiotherapy, The University of Queensland, St. Lucia, Brisbane, Queensland, Australia

Russell Volpe
Professor and Chairman, New York College of Podiatric Medicine, New York, USA

Justin Wernick
New York College of Podiatric Medicine, New York, USA

Foreword

In developing the objectives for the *Manual Therapy* journal it was considered important to produce a journal for the publication of scientific works in the field and at the same time have a special feature which focused on the clinical management of patients. Hence a Masterclass section was instituted where leading clinicians and researchers are invited to contribute work on aspects of contemporary clinical practice.

Peripheral joint dysfunction is commonly treated by musculoskeletal therapists in the clinical setting and therefore approximately half the Masterclasses presented in *Manual Therapy* have been concerned with examination, assessment and/or management of one or more peripheral joint dysfunctions.

This text is drawn from Masterclass articles published in *Manual Therapy* since its inception in 1995. The authors have been given the opportunity to update their original contribution using a postscript. The essence of a good Masterclass is that an expert in the field discusses a clinical issue and relevant examination, assessment, treatment and management strategies within the context of the best available supporting evidence for contemporary manual therapy practice.

This collection of papers includes 10 Masterclasses related to the peripheral joints. The authors of these papers are to be congratulated on their scholarly achievement which we hope will contribute further to contemporary clinical practice and clinical academic debate, and stimulate the formulation of yet to be answered research questions.

Items from a number of disciplines have been included in this Masterclass collection including podiatry, physiotherapy and chiropractic, emphasizing the multi-disciplinary nature of musculoskeletal therapy. The authors have addressed issues relating to current clinical concepts including dynamic stability, strapping and mobilizations with movement and have also considered a number of mobilizing and manipulative concepts relating to soft tissue and joint structures.

Karen Beeton, editor of the Masterclass section of *Manual Therapy* since its inception, has, over the years, facilitated the publication of a large number of Masterclasses. She is to be congratulated on coordinating the varied submissions and editing the entirety of the text. As co-editors of *Manual Therapy* we trust that clinicians will enjoy this series of papers and we look forward to Karen Beeton's continued work with *Manual Therapy* in the production of the Masterclass section in the years to come.

Ann P. Moore
Gwendolen A. Jull
Manual Therapy Editors

Preface

Manual Therapy is an international peer-reviewed journal that presents current research on all aspects of manual and manipulative therapy of relevance to clinicians, educators, researchers and students with an interest in this field. The journal, which is now in its 8th year of publication, includes review articles, original research papers, case reports, abstracts, book reviews and a bibliography. Such is the quality of the papers published, it is one of the few allied health journals to be indexed in Index Medicus and Medline.

One of the core components of the *Manual Therapy* journal is the Masterclass. The purpose of the Masterclass section is to describe in detail clinical aspects of patient management within a theoretical, evidence-based framework. This may relate to specific treatment techniques, a particular management strategy or the management of a specific clinical entity. Illustrations are a key aspect of the Masterclass in order to facilitate the integration of the clinical concepts by the reader. The authors are all leading clinicians and researchers in the manual therapy field. The Masterclass section of *Manual Therapy* journal provides an opportunity for these authors to present their approach to a wider audience. These Masterclasses therefore represent the cutting edge of clinical practice today.

Elsevier, the publishers of *Manual Therapy*, have decided to republish selected Masterclasses in two books. This book features a compilation of previously published Masterclasses focusing on the peripheral joints. The other book is a compilation of previous Masterclasses on the vertebral column. The purpose of this initiative was to draw together topics of related

interest and to facilitate accessibility of these articles for the reader. The Masterclass authors were invited to write a short postscript if they wished, reflecting on any developments in the evidence base and/or new developments in clinical practice since the original publication of their paper.

Manual Therapy Masterclasses — The Peripheral Joints consists of 10 Masterclasses on all aspects of assessment and management of the peripheral joints. The Masterclasses have been classified according to the regional areas including the shoulder, hip, knee and foot, and general topics of relevance for peripheral dysfunction. An index is included.

The postscripts which accompany the articles raise three issues. First, they demonstrate the breadth of research currently being carried out in the various fields and secondly, they draw on new evidence to support the use of the clinical concept or management strategy. Thirdly, they highlight the progression in the clinical reasoning and decision-making processes underpinning the concepts and the developments in clinical practice as a result of the increased knowledge base. In summary this collection of articles emphasizes that manual therapy practice today is not static but a vibrant, expanding and innovative area of practice that is moving forward and underpinned with a greater evidence base than ever before. This is so crucial in view of the drive today for all therapists to demonstrate evidence-based, efficient, effective practice.

It is hoped that, by bringing these clinically focused articles together in a book, it will become a valuable resource for clinicians when working in their practice or stimulate therapists when developing their own research interests. It is envisaged that it will also be an additional resource for undergraduate and post-graduate students exploring this field, as well as for educators. Manual therapists, whatever their professional background and area of work, are faced with challenges every day. It is hoped that these articles will enable them to draw on research-based, current practice so facilitating the achievement of the best possible outcome of care for patients.

The articles demonstrate the breadth of clinical practice available to therapists today. With the increasing emphasis placed on supporting clinical findings with research evidence this compilation of Masterclasses aims to fulfil that need.

Karen Beeton
Manual Therapy **Editorial Committee**

The Shoulder

SECTION CONTENTS

1

Dynamic stability of the scapula

S. L. Mottram

Kinetic Control, Southampton, UK

The ability to position and control movements of the scapula is essential for optimal upper limb function. The inability to achieve this stable base frequently accompanies the development of shoulder and upper limb pain and pathology. Unlike other joints the bony, capsular and ligamentous constraints are minimal at the scapulothoracic 'joint' so stability is dependent on active control. Clinically, it is noted that patients presenting with shoulder and arm symptoms demonstrate poor dynamic scapula control. Scapula setting is an exercise taught by physiotherapists to correct movement dysfunction associated with abnormal scapula positioning and dynamic control. Addressing the dynamic stabilization of the scapula is an essential part of the management of neuromusculoskeletal dysfunction of the shoulder girdle and an appropriate rehabilitation programme is necessary if this issue is to be addressed. *Manual Therapy* (1997) **2(3)**, 123–131

INTRODUCTION

Physiotherapists are becoming increasingly aware of the importance of understanding and addressing dynamic joint stability and muscle imbalance in the treatment of neuromusculoskeletal disorders (Richardson & Jull 1995; Lee 1996; McConnell 1996). The ability to position and control movements of the scapula is essential for normal upper limb function (Glousman et al 1988; Jobe & Pink 1993; Kamkar et al 1993; Wilk & Arrigo 1993). Shoulder girdle problems invariably present with a major component of movement dysfunction. It is recognized that an inability to control the movement of the scapula during activities involving the upper limb frequently accompanies the development of shoulder pain and pathology (Glousman et al 1988; Kamkar et al 1993). It is noted clinically that patients presenting with upper quarter dysfunction frequently demonstrate poor dynamic scapula control (Host 1995). The ability to assess movement function and correct movement dysfunction around the scapulothoracic joint is a key issue when addressing neuromusculoskeletal dysfunction in the shoulder girdle.

THE SHOULDER COMPLEX AND SCAPULOTHORACIC 'JOINT'

Consideration needs to be given to the anatomy and biomechanics of the scapulothoracic 'joint', the requirement for stability at this 'joint' and the mechanisms involved. The scapulothoracic 'joint' is a physiological joint between the anterior aspect of the scapula and the posterolateral aspect of the chest wall. It is not a true joint but the movement of the concave anterior surface of the scapula on the convex posterolateral surface of the thoracic cage (Williams 1995).

The shoulder complex (SC) is primarily concerned with the ability to place and control the position of the hand in front of the body (Peat 1986). As well as mobility, the SC needs stability during elevation, in order to give the muscles that move the glenohumeral joint a stable base from which to position the arm. The position of the scapula in relation to the chest wall is crucial for providing a stable base for movements of the upper limb.

The SC consists of the sternoclavicular and acromioclavicular joints (which link the upper extremity to the trunk), the scapulothoracic 'joint', the subacromial 'joint' (which is the physiological articulation between the coraco-acromial arch and head of humerus) and the glenohumeral joint. The sternoclavicular joint provides the only bony connection with the axial skeleton and, therefore, apart from this joint and the acromioclavicular joint the scapula is without attachment to the trunk.

ROLE OF THE SCAPULA

The scapula performs several functions contributing to stability and mobility of the SC. As well as a base for muscle attachments, appropriate orientation of the scapula optimizes the length–tension relationship of muscles associated with the SC; i.e. elevation of the acromion and the glenoid facilitates the optimum length–tension in the deltoid during shoulder abduction (Doody et al 1970; Hart & Carmichael 1985; van der Helm 1994). Rotator cuff function will be influenced by orientation of the glenoid (van der Helm 1994). The scapula provides the proximal articular surface of the glenohumeral joint. It orientates the glenoid to increase the range available to the upper limb, thereby increasing mobility. It also facilitates optimal contact with the humeral head, thus increasing joint congruency and stabilty (Saha 1971). The scapula upwardly rotates the acromion (i.e. lateral rotation of the scapula) allowing full abduction without impingement, which is vital to throwing or overhead activities (Kamkar 1993). The function of the scapula is dependent on the integrity of the acromioclavicular and sternoclavicular joints (Peat 1986). Full upward rotation of the glenoid during abduction lends mechanical stability to the shoulder by bringing the glenoid fossa directly under the head of the humerus (Lucas 1973). This also prevents impingement under the subacromial and coraco-acromial arch (Basmajian & Bazant 1959).

MOTION OF THE SCAPULA

The predominant movements of the scapula can be described as movements about a centre of rotation located in the scapula plane. These movements are upward (lateral) rotation; and downward (medial) rotation; elevation and depression; and protraction and retraction.

MUSCLES INFLUENCING SCAPULA POSITIONING, STABILITY AND MOVEMENT

The lack of ligamentous restraints at the scapulothoracic joint requires the muscles that attach the scapula to the thorax to have a major stabilizing role and hence these muscles need appropriate contractile and recruitment properties.

An individual muscle will have a specific action across this 'joint', but does not work in isolation. Trapezius and serratus anterior are the most important stability muscles acting upon the scapulothoracic joint. Johnson et al (1994) describe the anatomy of the trapezius muscle. The medial attachment of the trapezius muscle runs from the medial third of the superior nuchal line, the external occipital protuberance, the ligamentum nuchae, and the spinous processes and intervening supraspinous ligaments of C7–T12. The occipital and nuchal fibres pass downwards but mainly transversely to insert onto the lateral one-third of the clavicle. The middle fibres of trapezius run horizontally to attach to the inner border of the acromion and along the length of the crest of the scapula. Johnson et al (1994) refute the traditional view that the upper fibres of trapezius elevate the scapula as their fibre direction is predominantly transverse. It is proposed that the upper and middle fibres of trapezius draw the scapula and clavicle backwards or raise the scapula by rotating the clavicle about the sternoclavicular joint. This action would elevate the lateral end of the clavicle, rotate it backwards and cause upward rotation of the scapula. The fibres from C7–T1 and the lower half of the ligamentum nuchae are volumetrically the largest. During upward rotation of the scapula, these fibres do not significantly change in length; hence they maintain the horizontal and vertical equilibrium by stabilizing the scapula rather than producing movement. The inferior fibres ascend and converge to a tendon, which attaches to the tubercle on the inferior edge at the medial end of the spine of the scapula. These fibres upwardly rotate the scapula and resist the lateral displacement of the scapula from the pull of serratus anterior. These fibres work at a constant length. The scapula fibres of trapezius are especially active during the first 60°of abduction (van der Helm 1994), which indicates their role in maintaining good scapula position with initial humeral movement, and at 90° all fibres are active to counteract the pull of serratus anterior.

Serratus anterior is the major protractor of the shoulder girdle. Dysfunction of serratus anterior is demonstrated in patients with long thoracic nerve palsy. Typical features are winging (of the medial border) at rest, which is more prominent with protraction of the shoulder against resistance and downward rotation of the scapula from the unopposed action of the rhomboids and levator scapulae. There will be less lateral rotation of the inferior angle during abduction against resistance (White & Whitten 1993). There is, however, a lack of detailed studies on serratus anterior muscle alone.

Many texts agree that the upper fibres of trapezius, lower fibres of trapezius, and serratus anterior work as a force couple to produce upward rotation of the scapula (Palastanga et al 1994; Williams 1995). Johnson et al (1994) emphazise the role of serratus anterior. As serratus anterior draws the scapula laterally around the chest wall, the movement is controlled by the lower fibres of trapezius. In elevation, this force couple works to counteract the downward rotation force of deltoid on the scapula, and so maintains the optimal length–tension ratio in deltoid. This maintains the scapula in upward rotation, thus minimizing impingement and facilitating optimal glenohumeral congruency.

The muscle system has a function of providing stability. This is achieved by the regulation of muscle stiffness (Johansson et al 1991). The stability muscles involved need to be recruited prior to movement. This function has been demonstrated in lumbar stability, when transversus abdominis has been shown to be recruited prior to motion (Hodges & Richardson 1996). Although there is no experimental evidence of stability mechanisms about the shoulder girdle, it is hypothesized that the trapezius and serratus anterior co-contract to provide joint stability at the scapulothoracic 'joint'.

Muscles primarily involved in movement of the scapula are the levator scapulae, rhomboid major and minor, pectoralis minor and latissimus dorsi. Levator scapulae descends from C1–4 diagonally to insert on the medial superior angle of the scapula. Its action is to elevate, retract and downwardly rotate the scapula. It assists in scapula stability under load, but if it excessively dominates the scapula stability synergy, it will cause abnormal elevation and downward rotation. On dynamic movements it must lengthen to allow upward rotation of the scapula.

Rhomboid minor runs obliquely downwards and laterally from the lower ligamentum nuchae and vertebrae C7 and T1 to attach to the medial scapula border at the root of the spine of the scapula. Rhomboid major arises from vertebrae T2–5 and descends laterally to attach on the medial scapula border between the base of the spine of the scapula and the inferior angle. Their line of pull enables the rhomboids to retract and downwardly rotate but also elevate the scapula.

Pectoralis minor from the third, fourth and fifth ribs ascends laterally, converging to a tendon that inserts on the coracoid process of the scapula. This muscle exerts a strong pull on the coracoid process and can pull the scapula into protraction and downward rotation. Although in normal movement this muscle is not active during abduction or flexion (van der Helm 1994), if it is short or overactive it can maintain the scapula in an excessive protracted or downwardly rotated position. This is seen clinically with pseudowinging (Fig. 1.1).

Latissimus dorsi has an extensive proximal attachment including the thoracolumbar fascia. The muscle inserts onto the humerus but a slip to the inferior scapula angle may allow it to influence the scapula. If the scapulohumeral muscles, e.g. latissimus dorsi, infraspinatus or teres minor, become short or overactive they may pull the scapula into excessive abduction during arm elevation.

SCAPULOHUMERAL RHYTHM

The scapulothoracic joint contributes to both flexion and abduction of the humerus by upwardly rotating the glenoid fossa 60° from its resting position. During the initial 60° of flexion and 30° of abduction of the humerus, the scapula seeks a position of stability in relation to the humerus (Inman et al 1944), i.e. the motion occurs primarily at the glenohumeral joint. This illustrates the importance of the scapula being able to

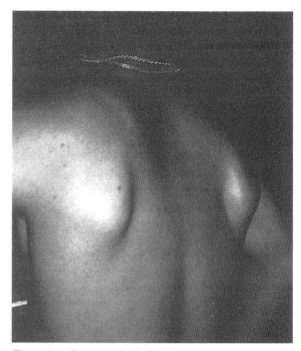

Figure 1.1 'Pseudo–winging' of the scapula. The inferior angle, rather than the medial border is prominent.

maintain a position of stability prior to movement. As the range of flexion and abduction increases, the scapula increases its motion until the late part of the range, when the movement is relatively minor (Freedman & Munro 1966; Doody et al 1970). During movements of the arm, the scapula needs to be relatively stable, but also upwardly rotate to allow full glenohumeral elevation. The ratio of glenohumeral joint to scapulothoracic joint movement and linearity of ratios is the subject of much discussion (Freedman & Munro 1966; Doody et al 1970; Saha 1971; Poppen & Walker 1976; Bagg & Forrest 1988; Michiels & Grevenstein 1995). Despite the obvious variability revealed in the literature, many anatomy textbooks continue to propose the 2:1 ratio of scapula to humeral movement based on findings by Inman et al in 1944 (Bagg & Forrest 1988). The degree of scapula rotation varies but the greatest relative amount of scapula rotation occurs between 80 and 140° of arm abduction (Bagg & Forrest 1988). Maintaining a stable upwardly rotated scapula is essential for normal SC movement, both in the setting phase and throughout the scapulo-humeral rhythm. This dynamic control of the scapula will ensure functional stability, i.e. the ability to control the translation of the scapulothoracic 'joint' during dynamic functional activity (Lephart & Henry 1995).

SCAPULA SETTING

Scapula setting is described as the dynamic orientation of the scapula in a position to optimize the position of the glenoid and so allow mobility and stability at the glenohumeral joint. The scapula is set in its ideal postural position — this is important both in the glenohumeral neutral position and elevation. This will involve isometric setting of the muscles that stabilize the scapula. The appropriate setting depends on muscle function and motor control. The ideal postural position of the scapula has yet to be clearly described and there is a need for further research in this area.

CLINICAL EXAMINATION

The clinical examination needs to identify any neuromusculoskeletal dysfunction and relate this dysfunction to the movement system. The movement system is the integrated and coordinated interaction of the articular, myofascial and neural systems of the body (Fig. 1.2). Each system needs to be examined and the influence of one system on the other considered. Faulty movement can induce pathology, not just be a result of it, so movement patterns need to be analysed in detail.

OBSERVATION

The normal scapula rest position has not been agreed upon (Sobush et al 1996), and this is probably because of the variation between individuals. However, there is general agreement that the scapula sits on the posterior thorax between the second and seventh ribs (Culham & Peat 1993; Williams 1995). The spine and scapula can be palpated to assess the relative positioning of the scapula. The optimum scapula position is

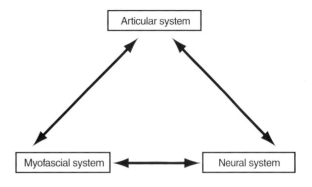

Figure 1.2 The movement system is an integrated and coordinated interaction of the articular, myofascial and neural systems of the body.

such that the superior angle of the scapula is level with the spinous processes of vertebra T2 or T3, the root of the spine of the scapula corresponding with the spinous processes of T3 or T4 and the inferior angle level with T7, T8 or T9, but it may be as low as T10 (Sobush et al 1996). It must be remembered that the scapula does not sit on the thorax in the frontal plane, but is angled 30° anterior to it (Peat 1986; Irrgang et al 1992). Observation of the scapula will identify its normal resting position. The ideal position should be in the normal rest position, which will not be at endrange but between elevation and depression, not in protraction but 30° from the frontal plane, in upward rotation and with the medial border and inferior angle flat against the chest wall. Clinically abnormal scapula positioning and poor dynamic stability is often associated with neuromusculoskeletal dysfunction. Kendall et al (1993) noted the importance of maintaining the upward rotation of the scapula and Basmajian and De Luca (1985) describe the normal scapula orientation at rest, with the glenoid in an upward position to enhance passive stability of the gleno-humeral joint. A typical dysfunction pattern is the scapula adopting a protracted and downwardly rotated position. Kibler (1991) noted the association of this posture with an impingement risk. Poor scapula stability mechanisms have been associated with increased laxity of the anterior glenohumeral structures because of increased stress on these structures (Glousman 1993; Jobe & Pink 1993; Kamkar et al 1993). With protraction and downward rotation of the scapula, the acromion drops forward and down and this can be observed (Fig. 1.3). Poor cervicothoracic and lumbar postures will enhance this inappropriate position (Fig. 1.4). Positions of the scapula may alter tension imparted on the upper limb neural tissue. Lack of muscular control may perpetuate postures, which add to irritation of neural tissue. A posture commonly adopted to relieve neural pathodynamics is protraction and elevation of the shoulder girdle and may involve activity of levator scapulae, upper trapezius and pectoralis minor.

PROPOSED MECHANISMS FOR FAULTY SCAPULA POSITIONING

If the scapula loses its stability mechanism, it typically adopts the postures described above. The stabilization function of stability muscles is influenced by postural changes, pain and pathology. Changes in the contractile properties of muscles and changes in connective tissue may influence muscle function. With disuse there is extensive atrophy of the tonic type I fibres and there may be length-associated changes (Goldspink & Williams 1992). These changes may influence the ability of the scapula stability muscles to maintain an ideal postural position of the scapula. Changes in the recruitment properties may influence muscle stability function. Pain can inhibit stability muscle function (Hides et al 1996), but joint pathology can inhibit muscle activity even in the absence of pain (Stokes & Young 1984). The latter is probably associated with changes in the afferent input to the central nervous system. Pain can increase the flexor reflex, which is seen clinically as spasm (Schaible & Grubb 1993). This spasm is seen in the movement muscles rather than the stabilizers and will have an effect on movement. Sensitized neural tissue may increase noxious input and set up inhibition and spasm. There is much discussion about the effect of injury and

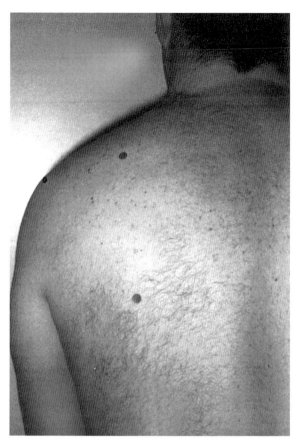

Figure 1.3 With protraction and downward rotation of the scapula, the acromion drops forward and down. The scapula is marked at the inferior angle, root of the spine of the scapula and the acromion.

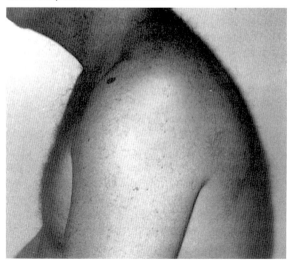

Figure 1.4 Poor cervicothoracic and lumbar postures will enhance a poor scapula position.

alteration of proprioceptive input. Damage to mechano-receptors will alter proprioceptive afferent activity and consequently a decrease in motor drive, leading to atrophy and weakness (Hurley 1997).

REHABILITATION PROGRAMME

The concept of improving proximal stability to allow distal function is now incorporated into shoulder rehabilitation programmes (Magarey & Jones 1992; Jobe & Pink 1993; Wilk & Arrigo 1993). Exercise programmes to improve scapula stability have been discussed (Magarey & Jones 1992; Moseley et al 1992; Ballantyne et al 1993), but they do not address the concept of setting the scapula in the ideal postural position prior to movement. Considering the physiological changes that occur with injury, disuse and disease, it is important to realign the scapula in its ideal postural position and recruit the stabilizing muscles to maintain this position.

SETTING THE SCAPULA IN THE IDEAL POSTURAL POSITION

Activation of the stability muscles in the ideal postural position is the primary aim of treatment. Initially the scapula position may not be ideal because of the length changes in the muscles and soft tissues or muscle inhibition, but the patient is taught to position the scapula towards the ideal position and perform an isometric contraction of the stability muscles — trapezius and serratus anterior. This is scapula setting (Fig. 1.5), the dynamic orientation of the scapula in order to optimize the position of the glenoid.

The scapula should be in its ideal postural position, not the inner range of lower trapezius, therefore 'drawing the scapula down and in' (retraction and depression) is not an appropriate command.

When considering scapula motion, it is important to visualize the action occurring in the scapula plane. With scapula upward rotation, the coracoid process moves upwards and the acromion backwards. The selection of muscles to

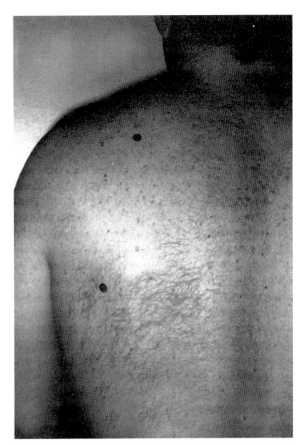

Figure 1.5 Setting the scapula in the ideal postural position.

be activated and the timing relative to each other is crucial for maintaining an appropriately positioned and stable scapula. It is important to ensure isolation of trapezius and serratus anterior and avoidance of substitution strategies. Once the scapula has been orientated in the ideal postural position, the stability muscles are consciously activated to maintain this position.

The patient must become aware of the ideal postural position of the scapula and this is optimized by the therapist. If the shoulder complex is in a protracted and downwardly rotated position, the weight of the upper limb must be unloaded passively. The scapula is orientated 15–30° forward of the coronal plane. With the scapula in this plane, the acromion and glenoid are lifted to upwardly rotate the scapula and the inferior angle moves laterally. The shoulder is allowed to relax in the direction of depression to the point where the inferior angle moves medially or the coracoid protracts. Once this position has been achieved, the patient must use low effort to maintain this position him/herself. A useful guide for re-educating stability muscles is to sustain a hold for 10 seconds, repeated 10 times (Richardson & Jull 1995).

Proprioceptive and feedback cues are important in improving scapula control, so appropriate facilitation techniques should be employed. It is useful if the patient understands the movements of the scapula. Observation of the path of the acromion is a primary cue (Fig. 1.6). Observing the coracoid moving away from the hand placed along the line of pectoralis minor can facilitate this movement (Fig. 1.7). Taping the scapula is a useful way of providing proprioceptive feedback (Host 1995). The aim of the tape is to

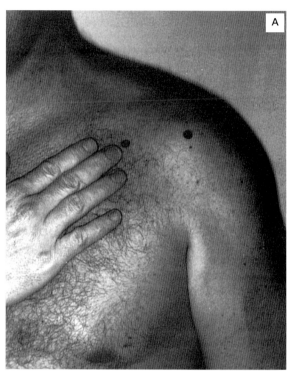

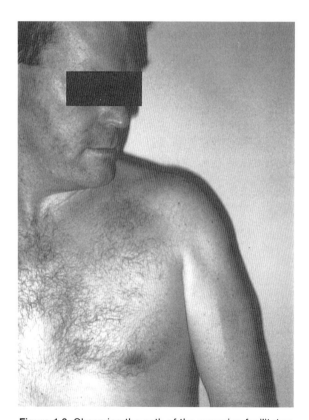

Figure 1.6 Observing the path of the acromion facilitates setting the scapula in the ideal postural position.

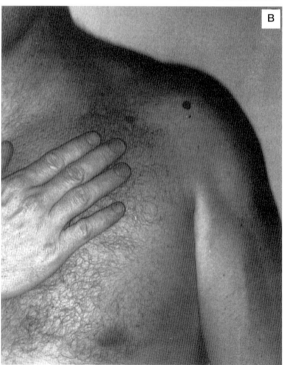

Figure 1.7 A & B Moving the coracoid process away from the hand placed along the line of pectoralis minor can be a useful facilitation technique.

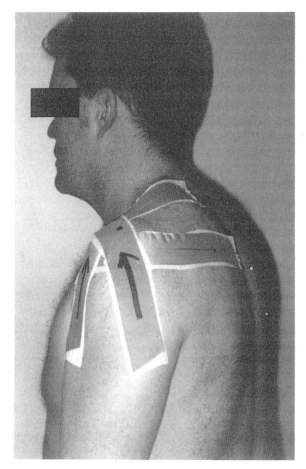

Figure 1.8 Taping the scapula is a useful way of providing proprioceptive feedback. The arrows indicate the line of pull of the tape to restore the scapula to its ideal postural position from a protracted and downwardly rotated position.

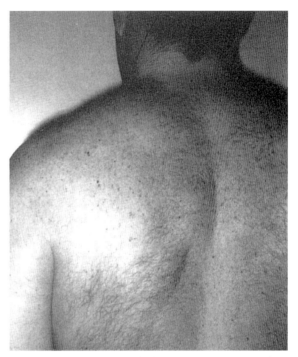

Figure 1.9 Common substitution strategies when setting the scapula include retraction with maximum depression, which downwardly rotates the scapula.

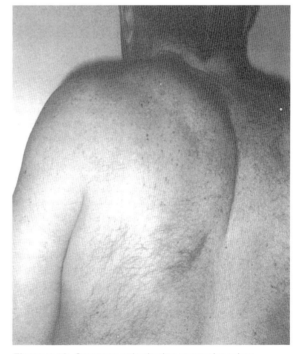

Figure 1.10 Common substitution strategies when setting the scapula include retraction with elevation.

position the scapula in the ideal postural position (Fig. 1.8).

It is important to avoid substitution strategies when setting the scapula. Common substitution strategies are:

1. Retraction with maximum depression which downwardly rotates the scapula (Fig. 1.9)
2. Retraction with elevation (Fig. 1.10)
3. Fixing the humerus to enable the scapulohumeral muscles (e.g. latissimus dorsi, teres minor, infraspinatus) to move the scapula instead of scapulothoracic muscles.

PROGRESSION

Once the appropriate scapula position has been achieved, it is important to regain dynamic control of the scapulothoracic joint. The scapula is set in its ideal postural position and maintained in this position using an isometric contraction of the stability muscles. The glenohumeral joint is flexed to 90° or abducted to 60° independently without scapulothoracic movement and with appropriate glenohumeral rotation (Fig. 1.11). The range of the humerus elevation is dictated by the control of the scapula. This exercise should be performed with low effort and with slow repetitions to facilitate the change in motor recruitment patterns. Once this dynamic control has been

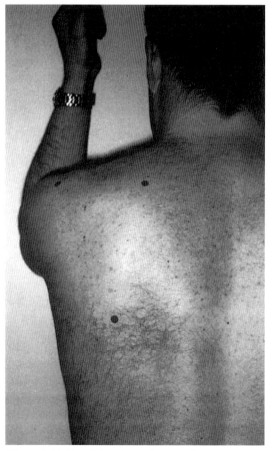

Figure 1.11 Regaining dynamic control once the set position has been achieved. The arm is flexed to 90° independently without scapulothoracic movement.

achieved, rehabilitation needs to be progressed to ensure normal scapulohumeral rhythm with overhead activities.

When dynamic control has been achieved, muscle imbalance issues must be addressed. The stabilizing muscles need appropriate control and recruitment to be able to hold the scapula in its ideal postural position under load. For an example of traditional muscle testing, reference should be made to Kendall et al (1993). An appropriate programme to achieve this control under load is as follows.

1. Scapula is set in the ideal postural position with the arm overhead.
2. Scapula is set in the ideal postural position with the arm overhead and a small range of lateral rotation of the shoulder–wrist lift (Fig. 1.12).
3. Scapula is set in the ideal postural position with the arm overhead and a small range of medial rotation of the shoulder–elbow lift.
4. Scapula is set in the ideal postural position with the arm overhead–short lever arm lift
5. Scapula is set in the ideal postural position with the arm overhead–long lever arm lift (Fig. 1.13).
6. Scapula is set in the ideal postural position with the arm overhead–long lever lifts with added weight.

The key points to consider when designing a programme are:

1. Initially the contraction force should be low (<30% maximum voluntary contraction) to ensure low-threshold tonic fibre recruitment.
2. The contraction should be sustained and repeated so as to improve the endurance properties of the muscle (Richardson & Jull 1995).

With increasing load (long limb lever) the contraction force must increase above 30% effort and co-activation of other synergists is acceptable provided the ideal postural position of the scapula is controlled.

Once the stability programme is progressing, active lengthening of the tight tissues can be targeted, remembering the ideal length of these

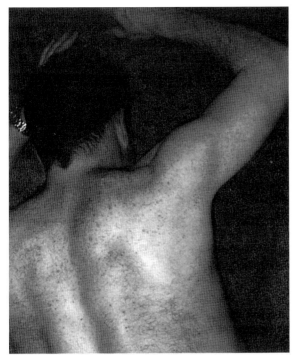

Figure 1.12 Regaining appropriate control and recruitment of stability muscles: with scapula set with arm overhead, small-range lateral rotation of the humerus–wrist lift is effected.

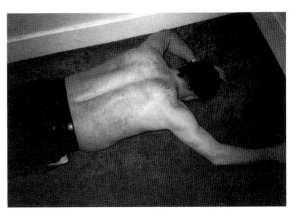

Figure 1.13 Regaining appropriate control and recruitment of stability muscles: scapula is set with arm overhead–arm lift with long lever.

muscles is necessary to allow ideal scapula movement (van de Helm 1994). Active lengthening should only be incorporated into the programme once the stability of the scapula has been regained. Techniques to address the abnormal afferent barrage from overactive muscles can be utilized at an early stage (Travell & Simons 1983; Gunn 1996).

Incorporated into this programme is dynamic postural retraining, by frequent tonic activation of the scapula stability muscles, into postural, functional, occupational, recreational and sporting activities. The facilitation of scapula stabilization optimizes SC function, but should not be used in isolation. Articular dysfunction, and neural and myofascial pathology, which are frequently concurrent or due to stability dysfunction, will need to be addressed.

REFERENCES

Bagg SD, Forrest WJ 1988 Electromyographic study of the scapula rotators during arm abduction in the scapula plane. American Journal of Physical Medicine 65(3): 111–124

Ballantyne BT, O'Hare SJ, Paschall JL et al 1993 Electromyographic activity of selected shoulder muscles in commonly used therapeutic exercises. Physical Therapy 73(10): 668–682

Basmajian JV, Bazant FJ 1959 Factors preventing downward dislocation of the adducted shoulder. Journal of Bone and Joint Surgery 41A: 1182–1186

Basmajian JV, De Luca CJ 1985 Muscles Alive — Their Function Revealed by Electromyography, 5th edn Williams & Wilkins, Baltimore, p273–276

Culham E, Peat M 1993 Functional anatomy of the shoulder complex. Journal of Orthopaedic Sports Physical Therapy 18(1): 342–350

Doody SG, Freedman L, Waterland JC 1970 Shoulder movements during abduction in the scapula plane. Archives of Physical Medicine and Rehabilitation 51: 595–604

Freedman L, Munro RR 1966 Abduction of the arm in the scapula plane: scapular and glenohumeral movements. Journal of Bone and Joint Surgery 48A(8): 1503–1510

Glousman R 1993 Electromyographic analysis and its role in the athletic shoulder. Clinical Orthopaedics and Related Research 288: 27–34

Glousman R, Jobe F, Tibone J, Moynes D, Antonelli D, Perry J 1988 Dynamic electromyographic analysis of the throwing shoulder with glenohumeral instability. Journal of Bone and Joint Surgery 70A: 220–226

Goldspink G, Williams PE 1992 Muscle fibre and connective tissue changes associated with use and disuse. In: Ada L, Canning C Key (eds) Issues in

Neurological Physiotherapy. Butterworth-Heinemann: Oxford, pp 197–218

Gunn CC 1996 The Gunn Approach to the Treatment of Chronic Pain; Intramuscular Stimulation for Myofascial Pain of Radiculopathic Origin, 2nd edn. Churchill Livingstone, Edinburgh, pp 3–19

Hart DL, Carmichael SW 1985 Biomechanics of the shoulder. Journal of Orthopaedic and Sports Physical Therapy 6(4): 229–234

Hides JA, Richardson CA, Jull GA 1996 Multifidus muscle recovery is not automatic after resolution of acute, first-episode low back pain. Spine 21(23): 2763–2769

Hodges PW, Richardson CA 1996 Inefficient muscular stabilization of the lumbar spine associated with low back pain. A motor control evaluation of transversus abdominis. Spine 21(22): 2640–2650

Host HH 1995 Scapula taping in the treatment of anterior shoulder impingement. Physical Therapy 75: 803–812

Hurley MV 1997 The effects of damage on muscle function, proprioception and rehabilitation. Manual Therapy 2(1): 11–17

Inman VT, Saunders JB, Abbot LC 1944 Observations on the function of the shoulder joint. Journal of Bone and Joint Surgery 26: 1–30

Irrgang JJ, Whitney SL, Harner CD 1992 Classification and treatment of shoulder dysfunction in the overhead athlete. Journal of Sports Rehabilitation 1: 197–222

Jobe FW, Pink M 1993 Classification and treatment of shoulder dysfunction in the overhead athlete. Journal of Orthopaedic and Sports Physiotherapy 18(2): 427–432

Johansson H, Sjolander P, Sojka P 1991 Receptors in the knee joint ligaments and their role in the biomechanics of the joint. Critical Reviews in Biomedical Engineering 18(5): 341–368

Johnson G, Bogduk N, Nowitzke A, House D 1994 Anatomy and actions of trapezius muscle. Clinical biomechanics 9: 44–50

Kamkar A, Irrang JJ, Whitney SL 1993 Nonoperative management of secondary shoulder impingement syndrome. Journal of Orthopaedic and Sports Physical Therapy 17(5): 212–224

Kendall FP, McCreary EK, Provance PG 1993 Muscles Testing & Function, 3rd edn. Williams & Wilkins, Baltimore, p.343

Kibler WB 1991 Role of the scapula in overhead throwing motion. Contemporary Orthopaedics 22(5): 525–533

Lee DG 1996 Rotational instability of the mid-thoracic spine: assessment and management. Manual Therapy 1(5): 234–241

Lephart SM, Henry TJ 1995 Functional rehabilitation for the upper and lower extremity. Orthopaedic Clinics of North America 26(3): 579–593

Lucas D 1973 Biomechanics of the shoulder joint. Archives of Surgery 107: 425–432

Magarey M, Jones M 1992 Clinical diagnosis and management of minor shoulder instabilities. Australian Journal of Physiotherapy 38: 269–280

McConnell J 1996 Management of patellofemoral problems. Manual Therapy 1(2): 60–66

Michiels I, Grevenstein J 1995 Kinematics of shoulder abduction in the scapula plane. Clinical Biomechanics 10(3): 137–143

Moseley JB, Jobe FW, Pink M, Perry J, Tibone J 1992 EMG analysis of the scapula muscles during a shoulder rehabilitation program. American Journal of Sports Medicine 20(2): 128–134

Palastanga N, Field D, Soames R 1994 Anatomy and Human Movement – Structure and Function, 2nd edn. Butterworth-Heinemann, Oxford, p.94

Peat M 1986 Functional anatomy of the shoulder complex. Physical Therapy 66(12): 1855–1865

Poppen N, Walker P 1976 Normal and abnormal motion of the shoulder. Journal of Bone and Joint Surgery 58A: 195–201

Richardson CA, Jull A 1995 Muscle control–pain control. What exercises would you prescribe? Manual Therapy 1(1): 1–9

Saha AK 1971 Dynamic stability of the glenohumeral joint. Acta Orthopaedica Scandinavica 42: 491–505

Schaible H, Grubb BD 1993 Afferent and spinal mechanisms of joint pain. Pain 55: 5–54

Sobush DC, Simoneau GG, Dietz KE, Levene JA, Grossman RE, Smith WB 1996 The Lennie Test for measuring scapula position in healthy young adult females: a reliability and validity study. Journal of Orthopaedic and Sports Physical Therapy 23(1): 39–50

Stokes M, Young A 1984 The contribution of reflex inhibition to arthrogenous muscle wasting. Clinical Science 67: 7–14

Travell JG, Simons DG 1983 Myofascial Pain and Dysfunction. The Trigger Point Manual — The Upper Extremities. Williams & Wilkins, Baltimore

van der Helm FCT 1994 Analysis of the kinematic and dynamic behavior of the shoulder mechanism. Journal of Biomechanics 27(5): 527–550

White S, Whitten C 1993 Long thoracic nerve palsy in a professional ballet dancer. American Journal of Sports Medicine 21(4): 626–628

Wilk KE, Arrigo C 1993 Current concepts in the rehabilitation of the athletic shoulder. Journal of Orthopaedic and Sports Physical Therapy 18(10): 365–378

Williams PL, ed 1995 Gray's Anatomy, 38th edn. Churchill Livingstone, Edinburgh

POSTSCRIPT

The understanding of movement and stability dysfunction has evolved over the last 5 years and the assessment and rehabilitation of scapula dysfunction has developed as a result. This postscript will focus on two issues, the assessment of the site and direction of scapula stability dysfunction and control of scapula neutral.

Pain in the cervical spine, shoulder girdle region and arm may have causes or contributing factors unrelated or indirectly related to movement and stability dysfunction. This postscript, however, will only consider dysfunction that is related to stability dysfunction. Stability dysfunction is defined as inefficient low-threshold recruitment of the local and global stability muscle systems (Comerford & Mottram 2001). This stability dysfunction can be described as uncontrolled movement or 'give'. Inefficient low-threshold control of the local stability system results in uncontrolled translational movement or loss of control of neutral. Inefficient low-threshold control of the global stability system affects physiological or functional movements. This site of 'give' is often the cause of pain and pathology and so it is of clinical importance to determine the location of this dysfunction.

STABILITY DYSFUNCTION

The direction of 'give' is diagnostic of the stability dysfunction. It relates to the direction of tissue (muscle, nerve, joint, connective tissue) stress or strain that is uncontrolled, and, therefore, to the direction of pain-producing movements. The direction of 'give' that relates to symptom provocation becomes the clinical priority. Table 1.1 illustrates the directions of 'give' at the scapula.

ASSESSMENT

An observation of active movements will suggest regions of relative flexibility (hypermobility) and stiffness (hypomobility) based upon observation of patterns of movement. Stability dysfunction

Table 1.1 Site and direction of scapula uncontrolled movement/'give'.

	Uncontrolled translational movement	Uncontrolled physiological movement
'Give'	Loss of control of neutral	Elevation/depression Forward tilt Downward rotation Abduction/adduction Winging

can be confirmed with tests to evaluate the control of the 'give'. A clinical rating system for the assessment and reassessment of stability dysfunction has been described (Comerford & Mottram 2001).

Tests for the site and direction of 'give' of the scapula (inefficient low-threshold recruitment) are detailed in Tables 1.2–1.5. These tests are designed to assess the ability of the subject to voluntarily prevent or control scapula movement in a specific direction whilst load is applied with arm movements. If the subject is unable to control scapula movements with low-threshold efficiency, stability dysfunction is identified. The stability dysfunction can be described by the site and direction of uncontrolled movement, e.g. scapula forward tilt. Rehabilitation is then focused on retraining the dynamic control of the uncontrolled movement/'give'. Efficient low-threshold recruitment of the local and global stability muscles is required to control the 'give' and move the arm.

CONTROL OF SCAPULA NEUTRAL

The scapula neutral position is the region where there is minimal support from the passive osteoligamentous system. Myofascial support is needed to control this neutral position, which is not the end of range of movement. The control of scapula neutral can be assessed using the clinical rating system (Comerford & Mottram 2002). Loss of control of scapula neutral is identified by the subject's inability to control the scapula neutral position with efficient low-threshold recruitment

Table 1.2 Scapula stability dysfunction test: flexion.

The scapula is positioned in a neutral starting position with the arm by the side. The subject is instructed to prevent scapula movement while the arm is actively flexed to 90°.
The direction of uncontrolled movement is noted.

Test (load)	Site	Direction of 'give'
Flexion (90°)	Scapula	Abduction
		Downward rotation
in standing		Forward tilt
		Elevation
		Winging

Table 1.3. Scapula stability dysfunction test: abduction.

The scapula is positioned in a neutral starting position with the arm by the side. The subject is instructed to prevent scapula movement while the arm is actively abducted to 60°.
The direction of uncontrolled movement is noted.

Test (load)	Site	Direction of 'give'
Abduction (60°)	Scapula	Abduction
		Downward rotation
in standing		Forward tilt
		Elevation
		Winging

Table 1.4 Scapula stability dysfunction test: lateral rotation.

The scapula is positioned in a neutral starting position with the arm by the side. The subject is instructed to prevent scapula movement while the arm is actively laterally rotated to 45°.
The direction of uncontrolled movement is noted.

Test (load)	Site	Direction of 'give'
Lateral rotation	Scapula	Retraction
(40–50°)		Loss of neutral
arm by side		Downward rotation
		Forward tilt
in standing		Elevation

Table 1.5 Scapula stability dysfunction test: medial rotation.

The scapula is positioned in a neutral starting position with the arm abducted to 90°. The subject is instructed to prevent scapula movement while the arm is actively medially rotated to 70°.
The direction of uncontrolled movement is noted.

Test (load)	Site	Direction of 'give'
Medial rotation (70°)	Scapula	Downward rotation
Abduction (90°)		Forward tilt
in supine		

of the stability muscles *(under low load — unloaded limbs and trunk)*.

This is assessed in different postures and positions. The stability muscles used to control scapula neutral are upper trapezius, mid and lower trapezius and serratus anterior. With primary shoulder dysfunction upper trapezius is rarely clinically short. A lengthened upper trapezius may contribute to stability dysfunction and may demonstrate signs of muscle strain. Overactivity can be associated with protective neural tissue (Edgar et al 1994) and there may be secondary signs in the cervical spine.

RETRAINING CONTROL OF SCAPULA NEUTRAL

Retraining control of scapula neutral, previously referred to as setting (Mottram 1997), requires rehabilitation of efficient low-level recruitment of the local stability muscles to control scapula neutral, and integration into function (local and global muscle co-activation). An exercise to bias for upper trapezius is illustrated in Figure 1.14, and for lower trapezius in Figure 1.15. A com-

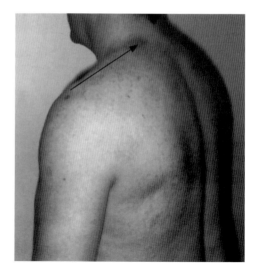

Figure 1.14 Control of scapula neutral: Upper trapezius bias: create transverse tension in upper trapezius — lateral clavicle towards cervicothoracic junction (Gibbons 2002, personal communication).

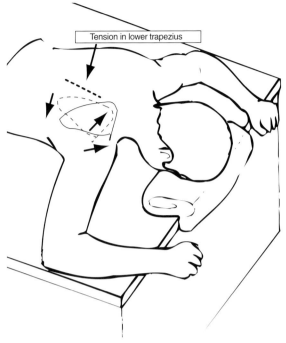

Figure 1.15 Control of scapula neutral: Lower trapezius bias; create tension in lower trapezius maintaining the scapula in a neutral position (controlling the inferior anterior glenoid). Adapted with permission from Comerford Physiotools.

mon dysfunction pattern seen with loss of scapula neutral is the positioning of the glenoid in an inferior anterior direction (inferior anterior glenoid (IAG)). This can be corrected by rotation: of the scapula in the coronal plane — observed by the acromion moving superiorly, while the inferior angle moves laterally (upward rotation); and rotation of the scapula in the sagittal plane, observed by the scapula moving upwards and backwards (posterior tilt); (Mottram & Woledge, personal communication), moving away from an IAG. Facilitation strategies for recruitment retraining include cognitive awareness; feedback; tactile, visual and technological; proprioceptive input and low-threshold co-activation of other stability muscles.

SUMMARY

Stability dysfunction at the scapula can be identified by the site and direction of 'give'. Further tests can identify local and global muscle system dysfunction (inefficient low-threshold recruitment). The author suggests that inefficient low-threshold recruitment requires retraining.

REFERENCES

Comerford MJ, Mottram SL 2001 Movement and stability dysfunction. Manual Therapy 6: 15–26
Comerford MJ, Mottram SL 2001 Functional stability re-training: principles and strategies for managing mechanical dysfunction. Manual Therapy 6(1): 3–14

Edgar D, Jull G, Sutton S 1994 The relationship between upper trapezius muscle length and upper quadrant neural tissue extensibility. Australian Journal of Physiotherapy 40: 99–103

2

Functional stability of the glenohumeral joint

S. A. Hess

Department of Physiotherapy, The University of
Queensland, Brisbane, Australia

Normal shoulder function is determined by the stability provided by the passive, active and control subsystems of the joint complex. Given the complexity of the shoulder, it is not surprising that it is one of the most common joints presenting with pathology. Knowledge and understanding of the anatomy and the intricate relationships of each of the subsystems is essential for successful assessment and treatment. This article presents a review of the anatomy, biomechanics and integrated function of the glenohumeral joint, which are essential for motion. The principles of rehabilitation of dynamic control of the glenohumeral joint are introduced. *Manual Therapy* (2000) **5(2)**, 63–71

INTRODUCTION

Normal function and stability of the shoulder is important for everyday life and is reliant on a balance between the muscular and capsuloligamentous structures. It is evident from the anatomy of the shoulder complex that the glenohumeral joint has little bony stability and hence many shoulder pathologies result. The shoulder complex consists of a series of articulations, numerous muscles and many ligaments, bursae and capsules. The anatomical joints include the glenohumeral joint, the acromioclavicular joint and the sternoclavicular joint. In addition, the scapulothoracic joint and the subacromial joint comprise the physiological joints. The glenohumeral joint is the centre of movement at the shoulder complex, with the acromioclavicular joint and the sternoclavicular joint extending the field of motion (Sarrafian 1988). While not minimizing the importance of all of the joints at the shoulder complex, the glenohumeral joint will be the focus of this article.

For clinicians, it is important to understand the mechanisms providing stability of the joints. Panjabi (1992) proposed a model to explain the stabilizing mechanisms of the spine, which appears to be well suited to the shoulder complex. Panjabi described three subsystems: passive (capsule and ligaments), active (muscle) and control (neural). These subsystems do not act alone, but are interdependent and thus create stability. In the shoulder, the articular geometry, capsuloligamentous structures, muscles and neural networks all contribute to its stability. The shape of the articulating surfaces and the capsuloligamentous structures are critical factors in determining the stability and range of movement available. These factors, in combination with muscle length and strength, play a major part in determining normal movement at the shoulder complex. Each of these anatomical structures is interdependent and intrinsically linked in function.

In order to successfully assess and treat pathology of the shoulder, an understanding of the anatomy and the interrelationship of its anatomical structures is essential.

PASSIVE SUBSYSTEM OF THE GLENOHUMERAL JOINT

The glenohumeral joint contributes the greatest range of motion to movement at the shoulder complex. It is a multi-axial ball and socket joint with the head of humerus being larger than the glenoid, so only part of the humerus is in contact with the glenoid at any orientation of the joint.

The glenoid articular surface is retroverted approximately 7°. It is suggested that this is important for maintaining stability and counteracting anterior displacement of the head of humerus (Saha 1971; Peat 1986). The glenoid labrum attaches around the margin of the glenoid fossa. There are differing opinions as to its importance in the stability of the joint. Lippitt and Matsen (1993) found removal of the labrum

resulted in increased instability of the humeral head on the glenoid. Sarrafian (1983) stated that the labrum did not deepen the joint substantially but more recent research by Howell and Galinat (1989) found the labrum deepened the articular surface by 50%. They propose it protects the edges of the bone and assists in joint lubrication. Peat (1986) suggests it may serve as an attachment for the glenohumeral ligaments. The shape of the labrum changes with rotation of the humeral head, adding flexibility to the edges of the fossa (Moseley & Overgaard 1962).

The capsuloligamentous structures reinforce the glenohumeral joint. The capsule is a lax structure allowing approximately 2 cm translation of the head of humerus in the resting position (Frame 1991; Pizzari et al 1999). On its own the capsule would contribute little to glenohumeral stability. Anteriorly, the glenohumeral ligaments and the attachment of the subscapularis tendon reinforce it. Posteriorly, the tendons of infraspinatus and teres minor strengthen the capsule. Inferiorly, the capsule has no reinforcing structures. Biomechanically, the orientation of the capsule has an influence on the motion available at the shoulder complex.

The superior glenohumeral ligament, coracohumeral ligament and supraspinatus aid in the prevention of downward displacement of the head of humerus. They also limit external rotation between 0 and 60° of elevation. The middle glenohumeral ligament is quite broad and lies under the subscapularis tendon, partly adhering to it (Saha 1971; Peat 1986). This section of the glenohumeral ligament is an important anterior stabilizer and limits external rotation from neutral to 90° abduction (Turkel et al 1981; Ovensen & Nielsen 1986; Ferrari 1990; Culham & Peat 1993). The inferior glenohumeral ligament attaches to the anterior, inferior and posterior aspects of the labrum and has thicker anterior and posterior sections with the inferior part being thinner. This section of the ligament limits elevation and protects the anterior joint in elevation. The posterior component of the inferior glenohumeral ligament stabilizes against posterior subluxation during elevation and internal rotation (O'Brien et al 1990; Culham & Peat 1993).

ACTIVE SUBSYSTEM OF THE GLENOHUMERAL JOINT

The glenohumeral muscles and their tendons comprise the active subsystem that generates stabilizing forces. As well as muscles that are primarily responsible for movement, such as latissimus dorsi, teres major and pectoralis major, there are muscles that play an important role in providing joint stability. This dynamic stability comes primarily from the rotator cuff, deltoid and the long head of biceps (Saha 1971; Peat 1986; Kronberg et al 1990).

The rotator cuff is the musculotendinous complex formed by the supraspinatus superiorly, the subscapularis anteriorly and the infraspinatus and teres minor posteriorly (Figs 2.1 & 2.2). The rotator cuff tendons blend with the joint capsule and are considered by some to be dynamic ligaments (Inman et al 1944). The tendons fuse into one continuous band near their insertions (Clarke & Harryman 1992; Minagawa et al 1998). This arrangement means that the effects of a contraction of one individual cuff muscle may not be isolated to that muscle but may influence the attachment of the neighbouring tendons (Soslowsky et al 1997). This finding becomes an important consideration during rehabilitation of the rotator cuff if any of the tendons have been torn or repaired. For example, activation of infraspinatus can result in tension in the supraspinatus tendon. This may be detrimental if the supraspinatus tendon has been repaired surgically.

The primary role of the rotator cuff muscles is to stabilize the head of humerus during activity of the upper limb. The contribution of the rotator cuff to shoulder stability may be due to contraction resulting in compression of the articular surfaces (Morrey & An 1990; Lippitt & Matsen 1993), co-contraction of the muscles causing translation of the head of humerus to the centre of the glenoid (Lippitt & Matsen 1993) (Fig. 2.3), activity producing joint motion that results in tightening of the passive capsuloligamentous restraints (Morrey & An 1990), the barrier effect of the contracted muscle (Symeonides 1972; Morrey & An

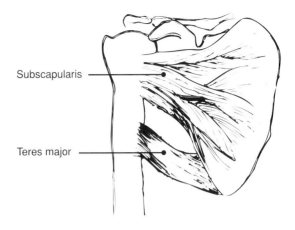

Figure 2.1 Anterior view of the rotator cuff.

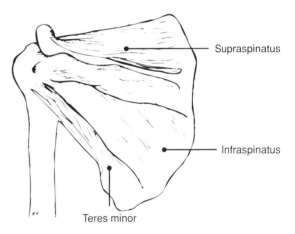

Figure 2.2 Posterior view of the rotator cuff.

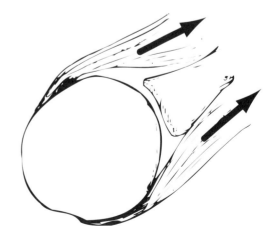

Figure 2.3 Co-contraction of the rotator cuff results in centring of the humeral head on the glenoid fossa.

1990) and passive muscle tension from the bulk effect of the muscles themselves (Ovesen & Nielson 1986; Morrey & An 1990). Ovesen and Nielson (1986) found an increase in the anterior and posterior translation of the humeral head when the shoulder muscles are eliminated, while Howell and Galinat (1989) found removal of muscle tissue allowed for increased inferior and superior translation.

Subscapularis activity is essential for joint stability. This muscle covers the costal aspect of the scapula and inserts on the lesser tuberosity of the humerus via a collagen-rich tendon (Fig. 2.1). The middle glenohumeral ligament and the origin of the anterior inferior glenohumeral ligament lie deep to the middle section of the tendon. The muscle has a large amount of collagen and has a role as a passive stabilizer, providing a barrier against anterior translation of the head of humerus (Symeonides 1972; Jobe 1990; Morrey & An 1990; Itoi et al 1996). Subscapularis functions as an internal rotator and a depressor of the humeral head but also has an important stabilizing action. It is common to see the head of humerus sitting anteriorly on the glenoid fossa due to tightness of the posterior capsule. Contraction of subscapularis will prevent further anterior and superior translation of the humeral head as the arm is moved and helps in the centring motion described by Lippitt and Matsen (1993). This will aid in the prevention of subacromial and posterosuperior glenoid impingement.

Infraspinatus originates on the infraspinatus fossa of the scapula and inserts on the greater tuberosity of the humerus (Fig. 2.2). Unlike subscapularis, infraspinatus is not excessively rich in collagen (Jobe 1990). It acts as an external rotator and a depressor of the humeral head. In addition, the role of infraspinatus may vary depending on the position of the glenohumeral joint. It has a stabilizing effect preventing posterior subluxation of the head of humerus in internal rotation, creating an anterior force by tightening the posterior structures. Cain et al (1987) proposed an additional role in preventing anterior translation during external rotation and abduction. During overhead activities, infraspinatus contracts eccentrically to prevent the distractive forces at the glenohumeral joint.

Teres minor arises on the middle portion of the lateral border of the scapula and inserts on the lower part of the greater tuberosity (Fig. 2.2). On its deep surface the tendon adheres to the posterior capsule. It acts with infraspinatus as an external rotator, providing 45% of the force (Jobe 1990).

Supraspinatus lies on the superior portion of the scapula in the supraspinatus fossa and inserts on the greater tuberosity (Fig. 2.2). It has an anterior and a posterior belly, which are proposed to function as discrete entities (Roh 1999). The anterior belly is larger, becoming the thick anterior section of the supraspinatus tendon. Conversely, the posterior belly is smaller and becomes the flat, thin posterior section of the tendon. It is postulated that the majority of supraspinatus tears occur in the anterior section of the tendon as the larger anterior muscle belly pulls through a proportionally smaller tendon area than the posterior section. Supraspinatus is active during any elevation activities and is important in stabilizing the head of humerus. It acts with the other rotator cuff, biceps and deltoid in torque production in the scapula plane. Research has been conducted on the rotational effects of electrical stimulation of supraspinatus. Ihashi et al (1998) found supraspinatus has external rotation and internal rotation actions depending on the shoulder position. In the lower ranges of abduction, with the arm in internal rotation, stimulation of the muscle produced further internal rotation of the humerus. In contrast, when the humerus was in neutral or externally rotated, external rotation was produced. As abduction increased, stimulation resulted in external rotation of the humerus.

The deltoid muscle has three heads arising from the distal third of the clavicle, the lateral acromion and the spine of the scapula, inserting on the deltoid tuberosity. The anterior and posterior deltoid components have parallel fibres and the middle third is multipennate. Elevation in the plane of the scapula is from the anterior and middle fibres with some action of the posterior fibres past 90°. The posterior fibres are more active in abduction. The deltoid contributes to approximately 50% of the torque of elevation.

Biceps brachii is active during elbow flexion and supination. It also has an important role to play at the shoulder. The two heads of biceps originate at the shoulder with the long head coming from the supraglenoid tubercle and the posterior superior glenoid labrum. The short head originates on the coracoid process lateral to the coracobrachialis. The muscle inserts laterally on to the posterior part of the tuberosity of the radius and the medial insertion is on the aponeurosis passing medially into the deep fascia of the muscles of the forearm. The long head of the biceps exits the shoulder through the capsule between the greater and lesser tuberosities into the bicipital groove. Anterior stability of the glenohumeral joint may be enhanced by the long head of the biceps. This may be achieved by limitation of external rotation through compression of the humeral head against the glenoid (Burkhead 1990; Rodosky et al 1994). During movement it should be remembered that the humeral head glides up and down on the tendon not the converse (Burkhead 1990).

While it is beneficial, in descriptive terms, to discuss the anatomy and actions of these muscles separately, functionally such independence does not occur. The importance of motor control lies in the coordinated contraction and relaxation of many muscles, not in the contraction of individual muscles (Zarins et al 1985).

BIOMECHANICS OF ELEVATION

The shoulder complex functions as a kinetic chain. Motion of the shoulder complex involves a balance of movement and muscle control from the lower limbs and spine all the way to the fingers (Kibler 1991). Recent research on pelvic stability has shown that movement at the shoulder is preceded by activity of the stability muscles in the pelvic region (Hodges & Richardson 1996). Although the shoulder complex comprises different segments, movement at any one of these may result in movement at another segment (Schenkman & Rugo De Cartaya 1987).

ARTHROKINEMATICS

The four articulations of the shoulder complex, the scapulothoracic, glenohumeral, acromioclavicular and sternoclavicular joints, may be described as individual entities, but it is the integration of these joints that is termed the 'scapulohumeral rhythm'. The interaction of these joints in a coordinated manner results in smooth movement of the shoulder complex. Elevation of the arm involves glenohumeral and scapula movement. Scapula movement is the result of motion at the acromioclavicular and sternoclavicular joints. The humerus rotates about the scapula at the glenohumeral joint, the scapula rotates about the clavicle at the acromioclavicular joint and the clavicle rotates about the sternum at the sternoclavicular joint (Schenkman & Rugo De Cartaya 1987).

When analyzing elevation, most movement occurs at the glenohumeral joint. There has been much discussion about the ratio of glenohumeral joint to scapulothoracic joint motion during elevation (Doody et al 1970; Saha 1971; Poppen & Walker 1976). Most literature still proposes the overall ratio of glenohumeral to scapulothoracic rotation being 2:1 with 120° elevation at the glenohumeral joint and 60° at the scapula (Inman et al 1944). McQuade and Smidt (1998) investigated the effects of load on the scapulohumeral rhythm. As the load increased, the scapulohumeral rhythm changed to a ratio of 4.5:1. It seems the scapula is providing a greater stabilizing force while the glenohumeral joint is moving.

External rotation of the humerus is considered to be 'obligatory' for maximum elevation. It has been theorized that external rotation allows clearance of the tuberosity posteriorly, preventing impingement on the coracoacromial arch. It may also release the inferior glenohumeral ligament to allow full elevation as well as to improve the articulation of the humeral head on the glenoid by rotating the head of humerus anteriorly (Morrey & An 1990).

ARTHROKINETICS

Although knowledge of the relevant arthokine
matics is important, understanding the forces
enabling movement of the joint articulations is
essential. Muscles almost always act in combinions
resulting in movement. Inman et al (1944) first
described the biomechanics of the muscles about
the shoulder with the use of electromyography.

The primary elevators of the glenohumeral
joint are considered to be the deltoid and
supraspinatus. This elevation is only made possible by the activity of subscapularis, infraspinatus
and teres minor providing a stabilizing effect
(Morrey & An 1990). All of these muscles act as
one of the important force couples at the shoulder
complex, the trapezius and serratus anterior acting as the other force couple producing upward
rotation of the scapula.

From 0° to 90°, the deltoid and the entire
rotator cuff are active, with deltoid activity
peaking at 110° and supraspinatus at 100°.
Supraspinatus activity decreases from this point.
Subscapularis is active in the initial phases of
elevation with decreasing activity after 130°.
Therefore, the ligamentous mechanism and tightening of the inferior capsule are important past
this point to provide anterior stability during
external rotation and elevation (Turkel et al 1981;
Morrey & An 1990). To complete full elevation,
external rotation is produced by infraspinatus and
teres minor, which remain active until the end of
elevation (Inman et al 1944; Kent 1971). Activity
of subscapularis during external rotation is essential in preventing impingement occurring if the
head of humerus is not centred on the glenoid.

Supraspinatus and deltoid have been found to
be equally responsible for generating torque
during arm elevation (Howell et al 1986). Since
most of the muscles acting at the glenohumeral
joint have a line of pull that is oblique to the plane
of the glenoid fossa, a combination of shearing
and compressive forces is produced. In the early
stages of elevation, the pull of the deltoid
produces an upward shear of the humeral head,
peaking at 60° of elevation (Poppen & Walker
1976). Contraction of subscapularis, infraspinatus
and teres minor counteract this by providing a
depressive action on the humeral head in the
glenoid (Fig. 2.4A). Subscapularis anteriorly and
the infraspinatus and teres minor posteriorly have
approximately equal cross-sectional area, so the
torque generated is balanced and represent a force
couple and also resists both anterior and
posterior translation of the humeral head (Morrey
& An 1990).

With continued elevation and change in joint
angle, by 90° the compressive forces are maximal
as the glenoid reactive force passes directly
through the glenohumeral joint, resulting in
compressive stability (Sarrafian 1983) (Fig. 2.4B).
Sharkey and Marder (1995) investigated the effect
of the loss of the rotator cuff on superior
migration of the humeral head during elevation
and concluded that glenohumeral joint motion
was not significantly affected so long as the
transverse force couple of infraspinatus, teres
minor and subscapularis was intact.

Interestingly, increasing the load on the arm
increases the activity in the rotator cuff more than
in the deltoid (Nieminen et al 1995).
Therapeutically, this demonstrates the importance
of the rotator cuff during activity and illustrates
the need to achieve good control of the rotator cuff
during rehabilitation.

CONTROL SUBSYSTEM

Coordination of the muscle action at the shoulder
is regulated by the neural subsystem described by
Panjabi (1992). This neural subsystem provides a
critical link between the active and passive
stabilizing mechanisms of the glenohumeral joint.
Proprioception plays an important role in
moderating the function of muscles. Intact
joint position sense enables joint stabilization
and appropriate muscle activation resulting in
smooth motion (Borsa et al 1994; Carpenter et al
1998). This fine motor coordination requires
afferent input from the mechanical receptors in the
rotator cuff muscles, tendons and joint capsule
(Carpenter et al 1998).

Guanche et al (1995) found the presence of
mechanoreceptors in the capsule, creating reflex
arcs via capsular afferent nerves, resulted in

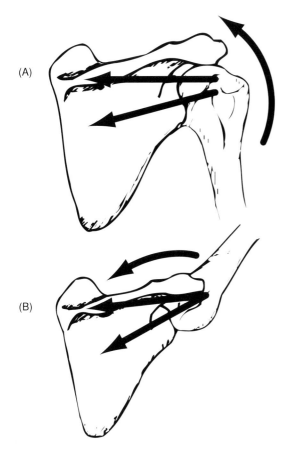

(A)

(B)

Figure 2.4 (A) Forces of the rotator cuff provide compression and depression to counteract the upward shear forces of the deltoid during early elevation. (B) Rotator cuff and deltoid provide increasing compression of the head of humerus on the glenoid as elevation progresses.

muscle contraction. Their research suggests that this may assist shoulder stability in humans.

With the intricacy of anatomy and biomechanics at the shoulder complex, the clinician must give consideration to proprioceptive mechanisms. For normal movement to occur, the joint position sense must be functioning.

REHABILIATION PROTOCOL FOR THE ROTATOR CUFF

The importance of therapeutic exercise for the treatment of shoulder dysfunction is now being recognized. To be effective in managing shoulder problems, it is essential to analyse the movement dysfunction and understand how the muscles will be acting. Research on muscle dysfunction in the lumbar spine has detected impairments in the muscle control that are linked to back pain, not muscle strength (Hodges & Richardson 1996). As clinicians, we can attempt to alter dysfunction of the active and control subsystems to improve motor control. This may prevent or alleviate problems with dynamic stability.

It must be remembered that scapulothoracic joint stability is an essential component of dynamic control of the shoulder complex. Exercise protocols to improve scapula stability have been discussed previously (Magarey & Jones 1992; Moseley et al 1992; Mottram 1997). Below is a management strategy aimed at improving the dynamic control of the glenohumeral joint.

This programme has been developed on the principle that isolated control must be achieved prior to progression into resistance, speed and functional rehabilitation.

PRINCIPLES FOR GAINING DYNAMIC STABILITY:

- Aiming for local control of the rotator cuff especially of inner range contractions
- Integrating and development of automatic control
- Gradually progressing into more unstable positions
- Control with additional load and speed requirement for functional retraining.

TECHNIQUES FOR GAINING LOCAL CONTROL OF THE ROTATOR CUFF

With all of the exercises, it is necessary to maintain scapula stability.

Conscious setting actions (centring humeral head)

These are commenced without additional load. Clinically, it is common for a patient to present with the head of humerus sitting anteriorly on the glenoid fossa (Fig. 2.5A). As discussed by

Lippitt and Matsen (1993), translation of the humeral head to the centre of the glenoid can be achieved by the rotator cuff. With palpation of the acromion and the humeral head, the patient is encouraged to use kinaesthetic awareness to draw the head of humerus posteriorly. The initial centring of the humeral head can be achieved in sitting or lying (Fig. 2.5B). These setting actions aid in the improvement of joint position sense and thus enhance more normal arthrokinematics.

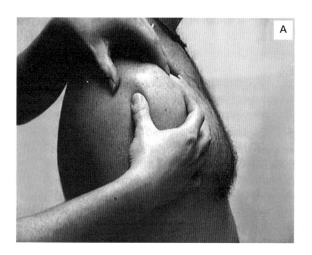

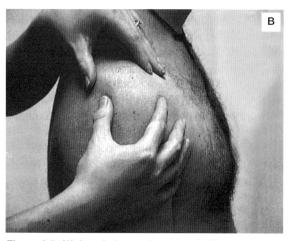

Figure 2.5 (A) Anteriorly translated head of humerus on the glenoid. (B) Active centring of the head of humerus on the glenoid with tactile facilitation.

Inner range holds of internal rotation and external rotation

Recently, Ihashi et al (1998) demonstrated internal rotation and external rotation will activate all of the rotator cuff musculature including supraspinatus. The arm can be taken actively or passively into the inner ranges of internal or external rotation and held in this position until fatigue occurs or substitution strategies are used.

Facilitatory techniques such as taping of the humeral head (Fig. 2.6), electromyographic biofeedback or tactile input such as palpation or sweep tapping may be utilized.

Joint compression through closed kinetic chain exercises

This encourages the co-contraction of both scapulothoracic and glenohumeral joint force couples. The starting position is critical with the patient maintaining neutral positions for the pelvis and shoulders. These may be commenced in sitting or against a wall with short or long lever arms, prior to progression into four point kneeling (Fig. 2.7).

INTEGRATION AND DEVELOPMENT OF AUTOMATIC CONTROL

Once local control of the glenohumeral joint has been achieved with a stable scapula, controlled movement of the glenohumeral joint should be encouraged. Patients with shoulder pathology often present with altered scapulohumeral rhythm. Clinically, it is often the case that once movement is initiated, the scapula is not stable and the rotator cuff musculature will reverse its origin and insertion roles, creating scapular movement and not glenohumeral joint motion.

Active internal and external rotation through range

By doing slow, controlled internal rotation and external rotation activities with a stable scapula, the rotator cuff will be providing stability and

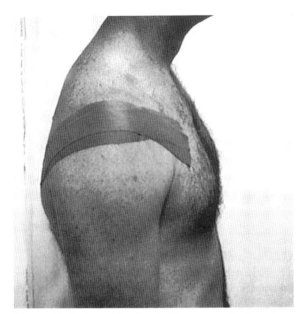

Figure 2.6 Taping of the head of humerus prior to active exercise.

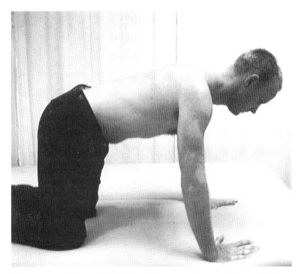

Figure 2.7 Closed kinetic chain exercises in four point kneeling — note the position of the shoulders and the pelvis.

movement at the glenohumeral joint not movement at the scapulothoracic joint. These exercises are started in neutral elevation and progressed into varying ranges of elevation once good control is attained. Commencing elevation activities in the plane of the scapula is often easier, as the muscles have a better biomechanical

advantage (Peat 1986). Once control is achieved, the movements may be performed with increasing speed.

PROGRESSIONS

Isometric contractions. Isometric contractions in all directions of elevation and rotation are started in neutral elevation with the humeral head centred and a stable scapula. The amount of resistance used is governed by the onset of any substitution strategies or pain provocation. Progression into elevation is then instituted.

Strength and resistance training for the rotator cuff

Active internal rotation and external rotation activities with resistance (e.g. tubing) are started in neutral elevation progressing into further elevation ranges (Fig. 2.8).

Closed kinetic chain exercises

Progression into more unstable positions using weight transfer, rhythmic stabilization, or balls or wobble boards is beneficial for retraining dynamic joint stabilization. Again, it is important to maintain good scapula and pelvic control.

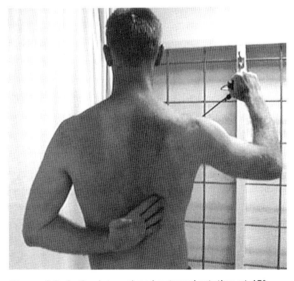

Figure 2.8 Active internal and external rotation at 45° elevation with patient monitoring scapula movement.

Combined movement patterns

These are useful for commencing functional retraining and should be activity or sport specific. Progressions with tubing, weights and speed are effective.

Advanced neuromuscular control

Wilk and Arrigo (1993) describe 'movement awareness drills' involving holds at the end of range and rhythmic stabilization drills which are beneficial for rehabilitation of the control subsystem. 'Flicks and wobbles' at the end of range and plyometric exercises, utilizing the stretch shortening cycle, are a good transition between strengthening activities prior to the return to sport or normal functional activities.

General strength training

These activities can be added to the programme as required once good control has been achieved. Gym programmes may be designed to strengthen muscles, such as latissimus dorsi and pectoralis major. Litchfield et al (1993) described some useful modifications to common gym exercises, which can decrease stresses on the shoulder (Table 2.1).

This programme has only addressed an exercise regime to achieve active control of a dynamically unstable glenohumeral joint. It must

Exercise	Modification
Bench press	Use a narrow grip
Supine chest flies	Standing flies with hands in view
Military press	Incline press with narrow grip
Lat pull downs behind head	Lat pull downs to chest

Table 2.1 Common gym exercises and modifications.

be remembered that once initial control of the joint has been achieved, lengthening of tight tissues should be targeted, as ideal length of muscles and capsuloligamentous structures is necessary to allow ideal movement patterns.

CONCLUSION

Each subsystem, although contributing to joint stability in a specific manner, acts in a coordinated fashion with the other subsystems, to create joint stability during movement. Disturbances in any of these systems can give rise to shoulder pathology. The shoulder region has always presented the clinician with many challenges. Evaluating and altering faulty mechanics of a particular shoulder movement may prevent a recurrence of symptoms. Understanding the normal biomechanics and the interrelationships of the anatomical structures of the shoulder is an important component of the successful assessment and treatment of shoulder pathology.

REFERENCES

Borsa P, Lephart S, Kocher M, Lephart S 1994 Functional assessment and rehabilitation of shoulder proprioception for glenohumeral instability. Journal of Sport Rehabilitation 3: 84–104

Burkhead WZ 1990 The biceps tendon. In: Rockwood C, Matsen F (eds) The Shoulder. W.B. Saunders Company, Philadelphia, pp791–833

Cain PR, Mutschler TA, Fu FH, Kwon LS 1987 Anterior stability of the glenohumeral joint. A dynamic model. American Journal of Sports Medicine 15(2): 144–148

Carpenter J, Blasier R, Pellizzon G 1998 The effects of muscle fatigue on shoulder joint position sense. American Journal of Sports Medicine 26(2): 262–265

Clarke J, Harryman D 1992 Tendons, ligaments and capsule of the rotator cuff. Journal of Bone and Joint Surgery 74A: 713–725

Culham E, Peat M 1993 Functional anatomy of the shoulder complex. Journal of Orthopaedic and Sports Physical Therapy 18(1): 342–350

Doody S, Waterland J, Freedman L 1970 Shoulder movements during abduction in the scapula plane. Archives of Physical Medicine and Rehabilitation 51: 594–604

Ferrari DA 1990 Capsular ligaments of the shoulder. Anatomical and functional study of the anterior superior capsule. American Journal of Sports Medicine 18(1): 20–24

Frame MK 1991 Anatomy and biomechanics of the Shoulder. In: Donatelli A (ed) Physical Therapy of the Shoulder, 2nd ed Churchill Livingstone, New York, pp1–16

Guanche C, Knatt T, Solomonow M, Lu Y, Baratta R 1995 The synergistic action of the capsule and the shoulder muscles. American Journal of Sports Medicine 23(3): 301–307

Hodges P, Richardson C 1996 Inefficient muscular stabilization of the lumbar spine associated with low back pain. A motor control evaluation of transversus abdominis. Spine 21(22): 2640–2650

Howell SM, Galinat BJ 1989 The glenoid-labral socket: A constrained articular surface. Clinical Orthopaedics 243: 122–125

Howell SM, Imobersteg M, Seger DH, Marone PJ 1986 Clarification of the role of the supraspinatus muscle in shoulder function. Journal of Bone and Joint Surgery 68A(3): 398–404

Ihashi K, Matsushita N, Yagi R, Handa Y 1998 Rotational action of the supraspinatus muscle on the shoulder joint. Journal of Electromyography and Kinesiology 8: 337–346

Inman VT, Saunders J, Abbot LC 1944 Observations on the function of the shoulder joint. Journal of Bone and Joint Surgery 26(1): 1–30

Itoi E, Hsu H, An K 1996 Biomechanical investigation of the glenohumeral joint. Journal of Shoulder and Elbow Surgery 5(5): 407–424

Jobe C 1990 Gross anatomy of the shoulder. In: Rockwood C, Matsen F (eds) The Shoulder. W.B. Saunders Company, Philadelphia, pp34–97

Kent BE 1971 Functional anatomy of the shoulder complex. Physical Therapy 51(8): 867–887

Kibler B 1991 The role of the scapula in the overhead throwing motion. Contemporary Orthopaedics 22(5): 525–532

Kronberg M, Nemeth G, Brostrom L 1990 Muscle activity and coordination in the normal shoulder. Clinical Orthopaedics 257: 76–85

Lippitt S, Matsen F 1993 Mechanisms of glenohumeral joint stability. Clinical Orthopaedics and Related Research 291: 20–28

Litchfield R, Hawkins R, Dillman C, Atkins J, Hagerman G 1993 Rehabilitation for the overhead athlete. Journal of Orthopaedic and Sports Physical Therapy 18(2): 433–441

Magarey M, Jones M 1992 Clinical diagnosis and management of minor shoulder instabilities. Australian Journal of Physiotherapy 38: 269–280

McQuade K, Smidt G 1998 Dynamic scapulohumeral rhythm: the effects of external resistance during elevation of the arm in the scapula plane. The Journal of Orthopaedic and Sports Physical Therapy 27(2): 125–133

Minagawa H, Itoi E, Konno N, Kido T, Sano A, Urayama M, Sato K 1998 Humeral attachment of the supraspinatus and infraspinatus tendons: an anatomic study. Arthroscopy: The Journal of Arthroscopic and Related Surgery 14(3): 302–306

Morrey BF, An K 1990 Biomechanics of the shoulder. In: Rockwood C, Matsen F (eds) The Shoulder. W. B. Saunders Company, Philadelphia, pp208–243

Moseley H, Overgaard B 1962 The anterior capsular mechanism in recurrent anterior dislocations of the shoulder: morphological and clinical studies with specific reference to the glenoid labrum and glenohumeral ligaments. The Journal of Bone and Joint Surgery 44B: 913–927

Moseley JB, Jobe FW, Pink M, Perry J, Tibone J 1992 EMG analysis of the scapula muscles during a shoulder rehabilitation program. American Journal of Sports Medicine 20(2): 128–134

Mottram S 1997 Dynamic stability of the scapula. Manual Therapy 2(3): 123–131

Nieminen H, Niemi J, Takala E, Viikari-Juntura E 1995 Load-sharing patterns in the shoulder during isometric flexion tasks. Journal of. Biomechanics 28(5): 555–566

O'Brien SJ, Neves MC, Arnoczky SP, Rozbruck SR, Dicarb EF, Warren RF, Schwartz R, Wickiewicz T 1990 The anatomy and histology of the inferior glenohumeral ligament complex of the shoulder. American Journal of Sports Medicine 18(5): 449–456

Ovesen J, Nielsen S 1986 Anterior and posterior shoulder instability: a cadaver study. Acta Orthopaedica Scandinavica 57: 324–327

Panjabi M 1992 The stabilising system of the spine. Part 1. Function, dysfunction, adaption and enhancement. Journal of Spinal Disorders 5(4): 383–389

Peat M 1986 Functional anatomy of the shoulder complex. Physical Therapy 66(12): 1855–1866

Pizzari T, Kolt G, Remedios L 1999 Measurement of anterior-to-posterior translation of the glenohumeral joint using the KT-1000. Journal of Orthopaedic and Sports Physical Therapy 29(10): 602–608

Poppen NK, Walker PS 1976 Normal and abnormal motion of the shoulder. Journal of Bone and Joint Surgery 58A(2): 195–201

Rodosky MK, Harner CD, Fu FH 1994 The role of the long head of biceps muscle and superior glenoid labrum in anterior stability of the shoulder. American Journal of Sports Medicine 22(1): 121–130

Roh M 1999 Anterior and posterior musculotendinous anatomy of the supraspinatus. www.medscape.com/Medscape/CNO/1999/ AAOS/02.07/07.roh-01.html

Saha AK 1971 Dynamic stability of the glenohumeral joint. Acta Orthopaedica Scandinavica 42: 491–505

Sarrafian SK 1983 Gross and functional anatomy of the shoulder. Clinical Orthopaedics and Related Research 173: 11–19

Sarrafian SK 1988 Gross anatomy and kinesiology. In: Post M (ed) The Shoulder. Surgical and Non Surgical Management. Lea & Febiger, Philadelphia

Schenkman M, Rugo De Cartaya V 1987 Kinesiology of the shoulder complex. Journal of Orthopaedic and Sports Physical Therapy 8(9): 438–450

Sharkey NA, Marder RA 1995 The rotator cuff opposes superior translation of the humeral head. The American Journal of Sports Medicine 23(3): 270–275

Soslowsky L, Carpenter J, Bucchieri J, Flatow E 1997 Biomechanics of the rotator cuff. Orthopedic Clinics of North America 28(1): 17–29

Symeonides PP 1972 The significance of the subscapularis muscle in the pathogenesis of recurrent anterior dislocation of the shoulder. Journal of Bone and Joint Surgery 54B(3): 476–483

Turkel SJ, Panio MW, Marshall JL, Girgis FG 1981 Stabilising glenohumeral joint. Journal of Bone and Joint Surgery 63A(8): 1208–1217

Wilk K, Arrigo C 1993 Current concepts in the rehabilitation of the athletic shoulder. Journal of Orthopaedic and Sports Physical Therapy 18(1): 365–378

Zarins B, Andrews J, Carson W 1985 Injuries to the Throwing Arm. W. B. Saunders Company, Philadelphia

POSTSCRIPT

The above article focused on exercise techniques to improve motor control of the glenohumeral joint. Patterning of contraction of the shoulder muscles was highlighted as particularly important during the rehabilitation process. It is important that physiotherapy treatment techniques, such as described in this article, are evidence based. Recent research in the area of motor control lends support to this approach to rehabilitation.

Research conducted at the Department of Physiotherapy, The University of Queensland, investigated the temporal patterning of the rotator cuff in overhead athletes with shoulder pathology (Hess et al 2000, 2002). A model of a reaction time task was developed to investigate the effect of pain on the shoulder muscles. Overhead athletes with shoulder pain and a group of matched control subjects performed rapid external rotation. This task was completed in sitting and in prone lying. The results demonstrated that the contraction of subscapularis was significantly delayed in the pain group ($p<0.0053$ sitting; $p<0.0446$ prone). In this pain group, latissimus dorsi was found to contract significantly earlier ($p<0.0001$ sitting; $p<0.0489$ prone).

These findings add weight to the clinical knowledge of the importance of the rotator cuff in maintaining the position of the head of humerus on the glenoid. Contraction of subscapularis prior to the contraction of supraspinatus and infraspinatus may enhance the centring of the humeral head on the glenoid as described in this article. This order of contraction of the rotator cuff may prevent the anterior translation of the humeral head often seen in shoulder pathology. It could be hypothesized that latissimus dorsi may be compensating for the inability of the rotator cuff to provide this centring.

Research has helped define the stages of rehabilitation. By following the principles for gaining dynamic stability outlined in this article, rehabilitation would address the research findings of the alteration of muscle patterning caused by shoulder pain. By initially aiming for local control of the rotator cuff, the delay in contraction of subscapularis with shoulder pain may be addressed. It is important to focus on the initial contraction of subscapularis and the centring of the humeral head on the glenoid, without the compensatory overactivity of latissimus dorsi. Following this, muscle activity must be integrated into automatic control and progressed into more unstable positions, with additional load and speed required for return to functional activity.

This research highlights the relevance of motor control in shoulder pathology. Physiotherapy should focus on evidence-based treatment techniques and rehabilitation must emphasize the patterning of contraction in an effort to prevent recurrences of shoulder pathology.

REFERENCES

Hess SA, Friis P, Myers P, Richardson C 2000 Pattern of contraction of the rotator cuff in throwers: A pilot study. Conference Proceedings: 2000 Pre-Olympic Congress. International Congress on Sport Science, Sports Medicine and Physical Education, Brisbane, p. 173

Hess SA, Richardson CA, Friis P, Lisle D, Myers P 2002 The effect of pain on the temporal patterning of the rotator cuff. Conference Proceedings: 2002 Australian Conference of Science and Medicine in Sport, Melbourne, p. 97

The Hip

3

Assessment and treatment of hip osteoarthritis: Implications for conservative management

K. J. Sims

Department of Physiotherapy, The University of Queensland, Brisbane, Australia

INTRODUCTION

The identification of factors leading to the development of hip osteoarthritis (OA), which are able to be influenced by physiotherapy procedures, was the focus of the previous article in *Manual Therapy* (Sims 1999). Treatment should be a logical extension of the assessment, which identifies the joint involved and the factors leading to the development of pathology. At the end of the clinical examination the clinician must answer the following questions:

- Is the hip involved?
- Is there a recognizable presentation of OA?
- What adverse mechanical conditions is the hip being subjected to?
- What is causing the adverse conditions?

The close relationship between the lumbar spine, sacroiliac joint (SIJ) and hip make differential diagnosis difficult. Lumbar spine and hip problems may often coexist (Offierski & MacNab 1983; Mellin 1988; Austin 1990; Greenwood et al 1998), and the SIJ may be associated with low back pain (Vleeming et al 1996) and hip pathology (Cibulka & Delitto 1993). The clinical reasoning process towards physical diagnosis and management is undertaken with a thorough history and physical examination. *Manual Therapy* (1999) **4(3)**, 136–144

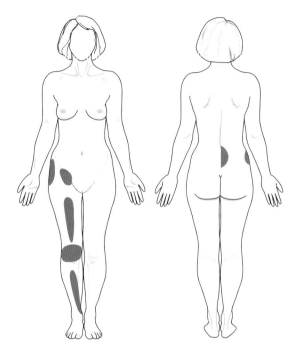

Figure 3.1 Typical pain patterns associated with hip OA (based on Wroblewski 1978).

CLINICAL EXAMINATION

The subjective examination is the first step in identifying possible hip involvement. The area of pain may provide some information (Fig. 3.1). Groin pain usually originates from the hip (Adams & Hamblen 1995). Buttock pain may arise from the SIJ (Fortin et al 1994), the hip (Wroblewski 1978) or the lumbar spine (Cyriax 1978; Apley & Solomon 1994). In some cases the only symptom of a hip problem may be knee pain (Adams & Hamblen 1995). Hip pain may be associated with sciatic-like symptoms (Grieve 1983). Clicking may be indicative of loose bodies or acetabular labrum tears (Fitzgerald 1995; McCarthy & Busconi 1995).

Hip pain is usually related to a particular movement or position of the hip joint, or the prolonged maintenance of a certain position. In many cases, stiffness after rest may be more troublesome than pain. Functional activities such as gait, gardening and driving may also aggravate hip symptoms. Past trauma or repetitive activity may also implicate hip pathology. The acetabular labrum may be damaged by even relatively minor trauma such as slipping or twisting (Fitzgerald 1995). Repetitive impacts may predispose to chondral damage or stress fractures. Recent immobilization, which may reduce the efficiency of the neuromuscular system, is a common clinical finding (e.g. from illness, or non-weight bearing related to a fracture in the lower limb). Childhood hip pain is relevant, particularly in males who are more at risk of developmental abnormalities (Wilson et al 1990).

The physical examination begins with a general observation of muscle tone, joint position, alignment and gait. The gait pattern may play a role in the development of the patient's hip disorder and must be analysed carefully (Sims 1999). Many gait and movement patterns may be related to abnormal motion in the lumbar spine and SIJ. Therefore, examination must always consider the influence of these regions on local hip mechanics, as well as possible sources of pain referral. In addition, increased motion in the foot may result in increased motion in the hip (Lafortune et al 1994). Functional tests such as squatting, and full rotation while standing on one leg, are also useful (Maitland 1991).

Visible wasting of muscles is common, in particular the gluteal muscles whose activity may be inhibited by tightness of anterior muscle groups (Janda 1978) or pain. Specific tests of hip abductor muscle function may also be useful such as the Trendelenberg test, (Hardcastle & Nade 1985), and the hip drop test (Sahrmann 1996). During the Trendelenberg test particular attention should be paid to movement of the trunk over the weight-bearing hip, as this provides a guide to the position of the centre of gravity. The implications of changes in the centre of gravity vector have been previously discussed (Sims 1999). The movement patterns of hip extension and abduction should be carefully analysed. The typical pattern of prone hip extension should be ipsilateral lumbar erector spinae, hamstring, contralateral lumbar erector spinae, tensor fascia lata (TFL) and gluteus maximus (GMax) (Vogt & Banzer 1997). This pattern of muscle activity may alter in the upright position. A delay in the activation of the GMax during prone hip extension has been reported following ankle sprain (Bullock-Saxton et al 1994). During hip abduction gluteus medius (GMed) and TFL should both be active simultaneously (Lewit 1991).

Inner range holding tests of hip extension (with knee flexed) have been used to examine GMax function (Richardson & Sims 1991) (Fig. 3.2) and inner range holds of hip abduction can also be used. The ability of tonic postural muscles to maintain a contraction in their shortened range against gravity is considered to be of fundamental importance in the development of motor control (Sullivan et al 1982). The modified Thomas test is used to evaluate the length of the hip flexors, abductors and adductors (Janda 1983). The prone knee bend test will also examine the length of the rectus femoris and evaluate the mechanosensitivity of the femoral nerve and lumbar plexus.

The examination of movement often reveals a capsular restriction, with internal rotation the most limited, and flexion, abduction and extension also affected. In very early cases of hip OA the first movement lost is internal rotation (Cyriax 1978). However, different presentations of hip OA may have different movement restrictions, especially in the early stage. Cyriax (1978) describes the loss of external rotation as rare, although many cases of hip OA appear to have a marked restriction in both internal and external rotation. A recent study of movement deficits in subjects with hip OA found little evidence to support the classically described capsular pattern (Bijl et al 1998).

Hip rotation should be examined in hip flexion and extension. The anterior capsule of the hip limits external rotation when the hip is in extension (Greene & Heckman 1994). During the movement examination, compensatory motions in the lumbar spine and pelvis may mask loss of hip motion and must be closely monitored by observation and palpation. For example, hip extension is often compensated for by extension of the lumbar spine. While examining hip motion, the clinician can also test for the presence of an acetabular labrum tear. The hip is held in full flexion, external rotation and abduction, and then moved into extension with internal rotation and adduction (Fitzgerald 1995). The production of the patient's pain (usually groin pain) or a click represents a positive test.

On some occasions, the pain experienced on some hip motions may be associated with excessive femoral head translation (caused by capsular tightness or muscular contraction). For example, the swelling out of the contracting TFL may cause a posterior translation of the femoral head. During hip flexion motions, tightness in the posterior capsule and piriformis may cause the hip to translate anteriorly. The clinician can recognize this phenomenon if the pain can be reduced by applying a translating force to the femoral head during the movement.

It has been contended that there is no accessory movement in the hip joint (Williams et al 1995). Whilst this may be true in the close packed position of the joint (extension, internal rotation, and slight abduction [Kaltenborn 1989]), it is possible to perceive three joint glides: in an A-P/P-A direction, in a mediolateral direction, and in a cephalad–caudad direction out of the close packed position (Figs 3.3 & 3.4). These tests should be routinely performed with the hip in approximately 20° of flexion to reduce tension in the capsule. They should then be repeated with the hip in greater extension to gauge the effect of

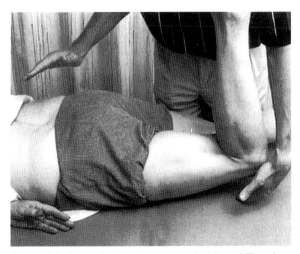

Figure 3.2 Assessing the inner range holding ability of gluteus maximus.

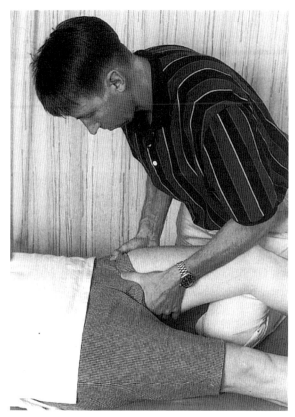

Figure 3.3 Examining the accessory movements in an AP–PA direction.

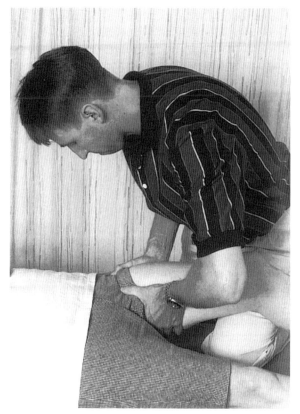

Figure 3.4 Examining the accessory movements in a mediolateral direction.

capsular tension on accessory motion. The accessory glides should also be tested in the patient's range of experiencing pain. The clinician should also compare joint accessory motion with physiological motion (Table 3.1).

In the early stages of degeneration, the accessory motions may help the clinician to identify the pattern of hip OA. In the migratory 'up and out' presentation, the longitudinal motion may be most restricted, whereas the medial migratory presentations may have a greater restriction on lateral glides. The A–P/P–A glide may be restricted in both presentations, or may reflect an increasing congruency within the joint. If the hip OA is relatively advanced or severe then all accessory motion may be very limited. In this case, the accessory glides will at least help in differentiating hip from lumbar spine and SIJ

pathology. The flexion adduction test remains a useful differentiating procedure when all other movements are pain free (Maitland 1991).

Table 3.1 Accessory motion of femoral head associated with physiological movement, based on Matles 1975 and Simoneau et al 1998. Neither paper clearly explains the basis of these results. If femoral head motion is influenced by the joint capsule in a similar manner to the humeral head, these motions may be mutually opposed.

Motion	Translation
External rotation	Anterior glide (hip in neutral)
	Superior glide (hip in 90° flexion)
Internal rotation	Posterior glide (hip in neutral)
	Inferior glide (hip in 90° flexion)
Abduction	Inferior glide (hip in neutral)
	Anterior glide (hip in 90° flexion)
Adduction	Superior glide (hip in neutral)
	Posterior glide (hip in 90° flexion)

It is often impossible to accurately predict the presentation of hip OA without an X-ray.

TREATMENT

The role of physiotherapy in the treatment of the hip is early recognition and implementation of preventative and curative strategies. Treatment should be a logical extension of the clinical reasoning applied in the examination, such that, having identified the hip as the source of pain, the clinician is also able to identify both the local and global factors contributing to the joint dysfunction. Local treatment includes the restoration of normal joint glides, the stretching of capsular and muscular restrictions and the restoration of normal neuromuscular function. Global treatment includes modification of gait patterns and activity, the use of a walking aid if necessary, and the restoration of normal joint motion and control in the SIJ and lumbar spine, knee, foot and ankle.

LOCAL TREATMENT

MANUAL THERAPY PRINCIPLES

Manual therapy procedures for hip joint OA require an understanding of the physiological effects of joint mobilization and the underlying disease process at the hip. Manual therapy causes a physical loading and unloading of joint cartilage, which facilitates the flow of synovial fluid within the joint, ensuring adequate nutrition for the articular cartilage (Twomey 1992). Research has shown that cartilage destruction occurs initially in the non-contact areas of the hip joint. The anterior surface of the periphery of the femoral head is a common site of non-contact cartilage lesions in the hip (Bullough et al 1973). This area will contact in internal rotation and adduction, which may explain the beneficial effects of the hip flexion–adduction technique. The use of joint mobilizations with compression (Maitland 1991) may also be very effective for stimulating synovial fluid flow. In the early stages of hip OA, simply improving cartilage nutrition may be a very important rationale behind the use of manual therapy techniques.

Manual therapy techniques should also facilitate improvements in joint range of motion, by restoring the normal accessory joint glides associated with movement. Two papers have discussed the directions of femoral head translation with movement (Matles 1975; Simoneau et al 1998) (Table 3.1). These translations are in agreement with the Kaltenborn Concept of the concave convex rule, which states that a convex joint surface (the head of the femur) glides opposite to the direction of movement of the bone (the femur) (Kaltenborn 1989). To this author's knowledge there has been no adequate *in vivo* study of femoral head translation with movement. Translation of the humeral head (a convex surface) occurs in the same direction as the movement of the humerus due to the dominant effect of the joint capsule (the 'capsular constraint mechanism') (Harryman et al 1990). A similar situation may occur in the hip as capsular tightness is a very common clinical finding. Hence mobilization of the femoral head in the direction opposite to the movement may be effective either by restoring the normal joint glide or by stretching the tight capsule.

Capsular tightness is recognized as an important predisposing factor in hip OA (Lloyd-Roberts 1955; Cameron & MacNab 1975), and many clinicians believe that early stretching of a tight capsule may prevent joint damage or at least slow further progression (Patla 1989; Hertling & Kessler 1990). Appropriate physiological and accessory movement examination should reveal the part of the capsule requiring stretching. However, stretching alone may be ineffective unless the question of why the tightness is present can be answered. It has been suggested that true capsular fibrosis cannot be overcome by manipulation, and if stretching helps it is because of its effect on the muscle (Gruebel-Lee 1983). This view supports the theory that muscles with capsular attachments can increase capsular tightness. The close relationship between the rectus femoris, TFL and the hip anterior capsule has been previously described (Sims 1999). In this case, stretching of the anterior capsule should also be accompanied by facilitation of the gluteal muscles to reduce overactivity in the anterior muscle group.

A treatment philosophy incorporating the different presentations of hip OA as part of the rationale for manual technique selection can assist in the development of a treatment plan. It can be hypothesized that the 'up and out' migratory presentation will respond better to techniques involving a longitudinal or medial-directed force and poorly to lateral distraction along the line of the neck of the femur. In contrast, the medial migratory presentations should respond better to a lateral distraction and be aggravated by a medial or compressive force. In the non-migratory forms both the superior and the concentric presentations may respond well to joint distraction. However, there are no guarantees of effectiveness of a technique, despite the best biomechanical or theoretical rationale, and so assessment of treatment effectiveness is vital.

The use of belts to assist in the application of techniques to the hip joint is widely advocated (Kaltenborn 1989; Mulligan 1996). The belt provides greater leverage to apply distractions, and can be used to support heavy limbs during the application of techniques. The use of gentle distraction forces in combination with joint glides may be very effective in restoring movement (Kaltenborn 1989). Mulligan (1996) has for many years combined joint glides with physiological motion and techniques involving compression and lateral or longitudinal distraction in combination with movement (Fig. 3.5). The belt in this case allows the operator to apply a glide and control a physiological movement simultaneously.

It is important to acknowledge that manual therapy procedures have wide-ranging effects that are not purely biomechanical. Gentler techniques may be very useful for pain modulation, or to facilitate lubrication within the joint, and may be equally effective as stronger belt or stretching techniques. The treatment of movement abnormalities in the SIJ and lumbar spine may also be necessary to improve hip function (see Lee 1989, for treatment approaches). In all cases manual therapy must be performed in conjunction with an effective exercise programme.

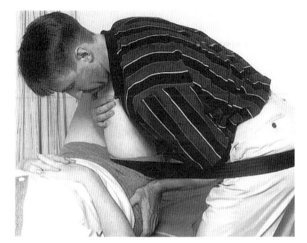

Figure 3.5 Applying a lateral distraction in combination with physiological internal rotation.

EXERCISE APPROACHES

Current knowledge indicates that the muscles about the pelvis most affected by hip pathology are the gluteals. These muscles have a tendency toward weakness and inhibition, whereas the TFL, rectus femoris, and adductors have a tendency to overactivity (Janda 1983). These clinical observations are supported by research which has found complete inhibition of gluteals and overactivity of the TFL and hip adductors in patients with hip OA (Long et al 1993).

PRINCIPLES

In order to encourage selective activation of weakened or inhibited gluteals, several principles should be followed. The gluteals are most active during the stance phase of gait, wherein they operate in their mid to shortened range. Hence, exercise should be performed in this functional range (Sullivan et al 1982). In the shortened range isometric contractions are considered to restore the stretch-sensitivity of the muscle spindle (Granit 1975). Effort and loading levels should initially be kept low to prevent overflow into other muscles (Kottke et al 1978). It has been suggested that skilled motor performance is characterized by selective inhibition of unwanted muscle activity rather than the activation of additional motor units (Basmajian 1977). Low loads, therefore, also allow the patient to concentrate on developing an awareness of the appropriate muscle contraction.

EARLY REHABILITATION

In the very early stages facilitation of the GMax may begin with static squeezes in a supine extension pattern. (Sullivan & Markos 1996). Small-range hip extensions in supine with the leg over the side of the bed (Carr & Shepherd 1982) are an excellent means of facilitating both GMax and GMed function (Fig. 3.6). This closed kinetic chain exercise is preferable to open chain exercise, such as prone hip extension, because the weight-bearing component effectively stimulates mechanoreceptors around the joint, thus improving muscular contraction (Dee 1969; Kisner &

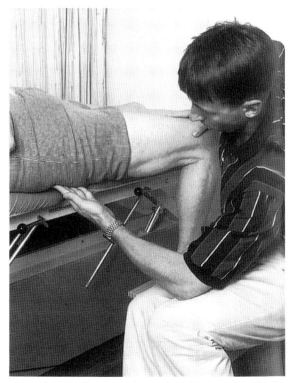

Figure 3.6 Facilitation of inner range hip extension in the early stages of treatment.

Colby 1996). Cutaneous stimulation of the soles of the feet is also thought to increase tone in the extensor muscles (Woollacott & Shumway-Cook 1995). Another benefit of this exercise is that it targets the inner range of hip extension, which is functionally important in upright stance.

The GMed can be exercised in its inner range in supine lying next to a wall. The patient gently abducts and externally rotates the leg against the wall, ensuring that GMed is being selectively activated by palpating it. The muscle can be preset by a gentle posterior tilt of the pelvis prior to movement. This exercise can also be performed in standing and, in this case, the GMed of the stance leg is being targeted.

Open chain exercises can be used if weight-bearing creates excessive pain. The GMed can be targeted specifically by performing abduction in side lying, but close attention must be paid to the precision of the movement. Weak or absent muscles can be compensated for by other muscle groups (Markhede & Stener 1981); thus abduction may be performed by TFL with no GMed activity. This can be minimized by not allowing the hip to drift into flexion, and by maintaining neutral hip rotation. A gentle active posterior tilt of the pelvis prior to the abduction movement is again a very effective means of targeting GMed.

In some cases it may be necessary to use lengthening procedures for overactive muscles before exercise can be done effectively. This will commonly involve lengthening the anterior structures such as the TFL, rectus femoris and underlying hip capsule. An effective method for this purpose is for the patient to be in a half-kneeling position and to then perform a posterior pelvic tilt. This usually produces a strong stretch in the anterolateral hip and thigh, which can be increased by a lateral flexion of the trunk to the opposite side. Care must be taken to ensure the patient is able to perform a posterior tilt of the pelvis correctly, as many will use a lumbar extension instead. This compensation is both ineffective and potentially harmful to the lumbar spine. It may also be helpful to provide feedback to the specific muscles being retrained. The use of electromyographic (EMG) biofeedback and facilitatory taping to the gluteals is a recommended means of providing feedback (McConnell 1995).

Even though a muscle may test as strong during manual muscle testing, there is no guarantee that the muscle will contract with the appropriate timing and coordination during movement patterns such as gait (Woollacott & Shumway-Cook 1995). Therefore, all patients should demonstrate an awareness of selective muscle activation before they progress to more advanced exercise programmes. Activities should be progressed so that the muscles are exercised as closely as possible to the way in which they normally function (Kisner & Colby 1996). Since most of the functional activities of the gluteals are performed in weight bearing, closed kinetic chain exercises are an appropriate choice.

PROGRESSION

The use of bridging exercises performed on the mat is one good method to improve strength and endurance. Bridging can be made progressively more difficult by reducing the base of support, increasing speed, and adding resistance. Controlling the lowering of the contralateral pelvis in standing will improve the eccentric control of the ipsilateral hip abductors. It is often easier to have the opposite leg supported on a chair to begin with. This is followed by standing with the opposite leg unsupported (Figs 3.7 & 3.8). Care must be taken to ensure precision of movement and both the lowering and raising of the contralateral pelvis is practised. A common substitution strategy is to use the contralateral trunk lateral flexors. This can be monitored with patient education, palpation, and EMG biofeedback. Progression is made by increasing the number of repetitions. When the previous exercise has been mastered, the patient can commence other activities, such as maintaining a contraction of the stance limb hip abductors whilst stepping the other leg through. This can be progressed by increasing speed, or adding resistance with theraband. To achieve good carryover from exercise to function, the therapist must ensure that the patient is aware of contracting the gluteals whilst walking. The patient can be instructed to overexaggerate the use of the gluteals whilst walking and to palpate the

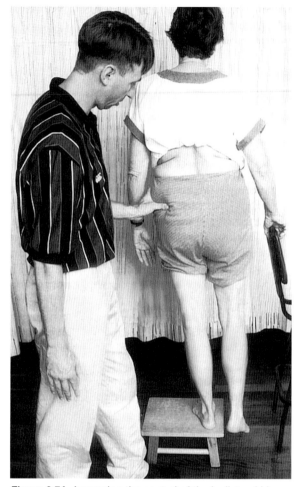

Figure 3.7A Improving the control of the ipsilateral hip abductors by raising and lowering the contralateral pelvis.

activity with their own hands. The patient should also attempt to walk as normally as possible, to reduce the potentially harmful effects of a limp (Sims 1999). This may only need explanation and demonstration by the therapist, or may require the use of mirrors or a video.

Single leg stance activities also have a role in retraining balance and proprioceptive awareness. There are many ways to further train balance, such as the use of balance boards, distractional tasks (e.g. keeping balanced whilst throwing a ball), and ball juggling. These should not be too difficult, as unskilled motor patterns will result in large amounts of muscular co-contraction

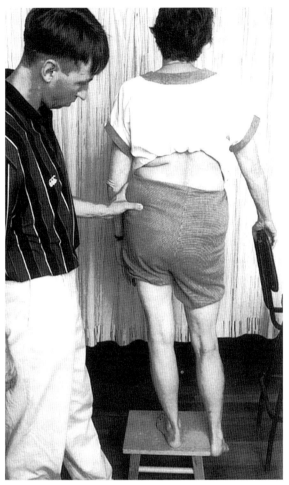

Figure 3.7B Improving the control of the ipsilateral hip abductors by raising and lowering the contralateral pelvis.

which may increase compressive forces on the hip joint. Balance activities should primarily be viewed as a means to facilitate muscle spindle sensitivity, and should, therefore, be followed by some of the more functional activities described above.

GLOBAL TREATMENT

The potentially harmful effects on the hip of altered gait patterns have been previously described (Sims 1999). The antalgic gait pattern is hypothesized to predispose the hip to an up and out migratory OA, and a Trendelenberg gait pattern may lead to a medial migratory OA (Strange 1965). The preceding section on exercise has described ways of improving local neuromuscular function, and discussed ways of improving the gait pattern. However, an altered gait pattern may have a multitude of causes including abnormal motion of the subtalar joint, the talocrural joint and the knee. These causative factors may need to be corrected by using talocrural joint mobilization, soft-tissue mobilization (e.g. of the gastroc–soleus complex) and orthotics to control excessive foot motion. It may also be necessary to retrain the eccentric function of the quadriceps to allow control of knee flexion at heel strike, which is crucial as a shock absorbing mechanism.

Any joint or muscle restriction that reduces the normal amount of lumbo-pelvic movement could have an impact on the position of the centre of gravity in single leg stance. The trunk should be displaced toward the stance limb in single leg stance (Perry 1992). A study has shown that patients with hip OA demonstrate a reduced amount of coronal plane motion of the pelvis (Thurston 1985). Treatments that improve lateral flexion of the lumbar spine using joint mobilization, or muscle-lengthening procedures for the quadratus lumborum, latissimus dorsi or lateral fascia lata, may improve the magnitude and direction of forces applied to the hip by allowing adequate displacement of the body weight vector toward the stance limb.

Dysfunctions of the SIJ may disrupt normal hip motion. For example, hip flexion involves a posterior rotation of the innominate bone (Lee 1989) and so a loss of posterior rotation may be a cause of hip flexion restriction. The same principles apply to hip extension, which may be limited by a lack of anterior innominate rotation. As many SIJ dysfunctions involve piriformis spasm, this may also reduce the range of hip rotation. In the older age group, exercise incorporating full pain-free range of movement in non-weight-bearing positions is important for maintaining cartilage health. Joint compressive forces can be minimized by the use of a walking stick in the contralateral hand, and carrying weights in the ipsilateral hand. These strategies reduce ipsilateral hip abductor muscle requirements and thus reduce compressive forces on the joint.

In summary, treatment of the hip requires an appreciation of the forces it is required to withstand, the local joint and muscle disorders, and the influence of the trunk and lower limb in the development of these disorders.

EVIDENCE OF TREATMENT EFFECTIVENESS

There are few published clinical trials on physical therapy management of hip osteoarthritis. A research paper that surveyed published trials of nonmedicinal or noninvasive therapies for the knee and hip was unable to find any data regarding the efficacy of exercise specifically for hip osteoarthritis (Puett & Griffin 1994). More recently, a randomized clinical trial of the effectiveness of exercise therapy for the hip has been conducted. Patients were treated with individual exercise programmes from physiotherapists and compared with those in a group who received education and medication from general practitioners. The main outcome measures were level of pain and observed disability. The results showed that the exercise group had a reduced level of pain and disability compared to the control group (Van-Baar et al 1998).

Another study has indicated successful pain relief for patients with hip pathology (predominantly OA) by the treatment of myofascial components of the hip and pelvis (Imamura et al 1998). Patients were treated with needling and infiltration of trigger points with lidocaine 1%, followed by physical therapy, home stretching and relaxation. The main outcome measures were level of pain (measured on the visual analogue scale), and pressure algometry. The design of this trial makes it difficult to determine which component of treatment had a beneficial effect and the physical therapy administered is not described. In addition there was no control group. There have been several single case studies of physiotherapy management of hip pain (King 1997; Sims 1998; Zimny 1998).

FUTURE DIRECTIONS

There is a need to incorporate the biomechanical and pathophysiological knowledge into appropriate physiotherapy management programmes for the hip. This article has outlined some treatment philosophies based on biomedical knowledge, but there is a gap in current knowledge on the associated neuromuscular disturbance associated with hip OA. Research into this area will provide direction for the development of the most appropriate exercise programmes, which are vital to maintain long-term improvements after the application of the many manual therapy techniques that have been advocated. The successful identification of hip neuromuscular dysfunction will also provide another outcome measure that may be used in clinical trials.

There have been few trials to determine the effect of physical therapy in the treatment of hip disorders. They are needed to identify the effectiveness of exercise and manual therapy. They are also needed to determine whether some specific groups of patients suffering from hip OA respond better to physiotherapy than others. For example those with a primary capsular restriction (e.g. 'up and out' migratory pattern) may be treated more successfully than those with bilateral hip OA associated with obesity. The future challenge for all physiotherapists is to prove that their services are an effective means of treating hip disorders. To ensure their effectiveness they must root manual therapy treatments in sound theoretical rationale and seek to increase the knowledge base of neuromuscular dysfunction in the hip. This will provide a balanced platform from which to manage hip OA.

REFERENCES

Adams JC, Hamblen D 1995 Outline of Orthopaedics, 12th edn. Churchill Livingstone, Edinburgh, pp 282–324

Apley A, Solomon L 1994 Concise System of Orthopaedics and Fractures, 2nd edn. Butterworth–Heinemann, Oxford, pp 174–193

Austin R 1990 Spinal lesions simulating hip joint disorders. Clinical Rheumatology 9: 414–420

Basmajian J 1977 Motor learning and control: a working hypothesis. Archives of Physical and Medical Rehabilitation 58: 38–41

Bijl D, Dekker J, Van Baar M, Oostendorp RA, Lemmens AM, Bijlsma JW, Voorn TB 1998 Validity of Cyriax's concept capsular pattern for the diagnosis of osteoarthritis of hip and/or knee. Scandinavian Journal of Rheumatology 27: 347–351

Bullock-Saxton J, Janda V, Bullock M 1994 The influence of ankle sprain injury on muscle activation during hip extension. International Journal of Sports Medicine 15: 330–334

Bullough P, Goodfellow J, O'Connor J 1973 The relationship between degenerative changes and load bearing in the human hip. Journal of Bone and Joint Surgery 55B: 746–758

Cameron H, MacNab I 1975 Observations on osteoarthritis of the hip joint. Clinical Orthopaedics and Related Research 108: 31–40

Carr J, Shepherd R 1982 A Motor Relearning Program for Stroke. Heinemann, London, p.107

Cibulka M, Delitto A 1993 A comparison of two different methods to treat hip pain in runners. Journal of Orthopaedic and Sports Physical Therapy 17: 172–176

Cyriax J 1978 Textbook of Orthopaedic Medicine, 7th edn, Vol 1. Bailliere Tindall, London, pp 594–621

Dee R 1969 Structure and function of hip joint innervation. Annals of the Royal College of Surgeons of England 45: 357–374

Fitzgerald R 1995 Acetabular labral tears. Clinical Orthopaedics and Related Research 311: 60–68

Fortin J, April C, Ponthieux B, Pier J 1994 Sacroiliac joint: pain referral maps upon applying a new injection/arthrography technique. Part II: Clinical evaluation. Spine 19: 1483–1489

Granit R 1975 The functional role of the muscle spindles—facts and hypotheses. Brain 98: 531–556

Greene W, Heckman J 1994 The Clinical Measurement of Joint Motion. American Academy of Orthopaedic Surgeons, Rosemount, Illinois, p. 101

Greenwood M, Erhard R, Jones D 1998 Differential diagnosis of the hip versus lumbar spine: five case reports. Journal of Orthopaedic and Sports Physical Therapy 27: 308–315

Grieve G 1983 The hip. Physiotherapy 69: 196–204

Gruebel-Lee D 1983 Disorders of the Hip. JB Lippincott, Philadelphia, p. 76

Hardcastle P, Nade S 1985 The significance of the trendelenberg test. Journal of Bone and Joint Surgery 67B: 741–746

Harryman D, Sidles J, Clark J, McQuade K, Gibb T, Matsen F 1990 Translation of the humeral head on the glenoid with passive glenohumeral motion. Journal of Bone and Joint Surgery 72A: 1334–1343

Hertling D, Kessler R 1990 The Hip. In: Hertling D, Kessler R (eds) Management of Common Musculoskeletal Disorders. JB Lippincott, Philadelphia, pp 272–297

Imamura S, Riberto M, Fischer A, Imamura M, Kaziyama H, Teixeira M 1998 Successful pain relief by treatment of myofascial components in patients with hip pathology scheduled for total hip replacement. Journal of Musculoskeletal Pain 6: 73–89

Janda V 1978 Muscles, central nervous motor regulation and back problems. In: Korr I (ed) The Neurobiologic Mechanisms in Manipulative Therapy. Plenum Press, New York, pp 27–41

Janda V 1983 Muscle Function Testing. Butterworths, London, p. 226

Kaltenborn F 1989 Manual Mobilisation of the Extremity Joints, 4th edn. Olaf Norlis Bokhandel, Oslo, pp 27–47

King L 1997 Physical therapy management of hip osteoarthritis prior to total hip arthroplasty. Journal of Orthopaedic and Sports Physical Therapy 26(1): 35–38

Kisner C, Colby L 1996 Therapeutic exercise—Foundations & techniques, 3rd edn. FA Davis Co., Philadelphia, p. 68

Kottke F, Halpern D, Easton J, Ozel A, Burrill C 1978 The training of coordination. Archives of Physical Medicine and Rehabilitation 59: 567–572

Lafortune M, Cavanagh P, Sommer H, Kalenak A 1994 Foot inversion-eversion and knee kinematics during walking. Journal of Orthopaedic Research 12: 412–420

Lee D 1989 The Pelvic Girdle: An Approach to the Examination and Treatment of the Lumbo-pelvic-hip Region. Churchill Livingstone, Edinburgh

Lewit K 1991 Manipulative Therapy in Rehabilitation of the Locomotor System, 2nd edn. Butterworth—Heinemann, Oxford, p. 111

Lloyd-Roberts G 1955 Osteoarthritis of the hip. A study of the clinical pathology. Journal of Bone and Joint Surgery 37B: 8–47

Long W, Dorr L, Healy B, Perry J 1993 Functional recovery of noncemented total hip arthroplasty. Clinical Orthopaedics and Related Research 288: 73–77

Maitland G 1991 Peripheral Manipulation, 3rd edn. Butterworth-Heinemann, London, pp 221–238

Markhede G, Stener B 1981 Function after removal of various hip and thigh muscles for extirpation of tumors. Acta Orthopaedica Scandinavica 52: 373–395

Matles A 1975 Motion of the hip joint. Bulletin of the Hospital for Joint Diseases 36: 170–176

McCarthy J, Busconi B 1995 The role of hip arthroscopy in the diagnosis and treatment of hip disease. Orthopedics 18: 753–756

McConnell J 1995 Lower Limb Biomechanics, Course Notes

Mellin G 1988 Correlations of hip mobility with degree of back pain and lumbar spinal mobility in chronic low back pain patients. Spine 13: 668–670

Mulligan B 1996 Mobilisations with movement for the hip joint to restore internal rotation and flexion. Journal of Manual and Manipulative Therapy 4: 35–36

Offierski C, MacNab I 1983 Hip-spine syndrome. Spine 8: 316–321

Patla C 1989 Lower Extremity. In: Payton O, DiFabio R, Paris S, Protas E, VanSant A (eds) Manual of Physical Therapy. Churchill Livingstone, New York, pp 477–483

Perry J 1992 Gait Analysis, 1st edn. Slack, Thorofare, New Jersey

Puett D, Griffin M 1994 Published trials of nonmedicinal and noninvasive therapies for hip and knee osteoarthritis. Annals of Internal Medicine 121: 133–140

Richardson C, Sims K 1991 An inner range holding contraction: an objective measure of stabilising function of an antigravity muscle. 11th International Congress World Confederation of Physical Therapy, London, p. 829

Sahrmann S 1996 Diagnosis and Treatment of Movement Related Pain Syndromes Associated with Muscle and Movement Imbalances. Washington University of Medicine, St Louis

Simoneau G, Hoenig K, Lepley J, Papanek P 1998 Influence of hip position and gender on active hip internal and external rotation. Journal of Orthopaedic and Sports Physical Therapy 28: 158–164

Sims K 1998 Grave's, gravity and the groin: a case study. Manual Therapy 3: 159–161

Sims K 1999 The development of hip osteoarthritis: implications for conservative management. Manual Therapy 4: 127–135

Strange FSC 1965 The Hip. William Heinemann Medical Books, London, p 226–262

Sullivan P, Markos P 1996 Clinical Procedures in Therapeutic Exercise, 2nd edn. Appleton and Lange, Stamford, Connecticut, p. 30

Sullivan P, Markos P, Minor M 1982 An Integrated Approach to Therapeutic Exercise—Theory and Clinical Application. Reston Publishing Company, Reston, Virginia, p. 27

Thurston A 1985 Spinal and pelvic kinematics in osteoarthrosis of the hip joint. Spine 10: 467–471

Twomey L 1992 A rationale for the treatment of back pain and joint pain by manual therapy. Physical Therapy 72: 885–892

Van-Baar M, Dekker J, Oostendorp R, Bijl D, Voorn TB, Lemmens AM Bijlsma JW 1998 The effectiveness of exercise therapy in patients with osteoarthritis of the hip or knee: a randomized clinical trial. Journal of Rheumatology 25(12): 2432–2439

Vleeming A, Pool-Goudzwaard A, Hammudoghlu D, Stoechart R, Snijders C, Mens J 1996 The function of the long dorsal sacroiliac ligament. Spine 21: 556–562

Vogt L, Banzer W 1997 Dynamic testing of the motor stereotype in prone hip extension from the neutral position. Clinical Biomechanics 12: 122–127

Williams P, Bannister L 1995 In: Berry M, Collins P, Dyson M, Dussek J, Ferguson M (eds) Gray's Anatomy, 38th edn. Churchill Livingstone, Edinburgh, p. 688

Wilson M, Michet C, Ilstrup D, Melton L 1990 Idiopathic symptomatic osteoarthritis of the hip and knee: a population-based incidence study. Mayo Clinic Proceedings 65: 1214–1221

Woollacott M, Shumway-Cook A 1995 Motor Control–Theory and Practical Applications. Williams and Wilkins, Baltimore

Wroblewski B 1978 Pain in osteoarthrosis of the hip. The Practitioner 140: 1315

Zimny NJ 1998 Clinical measuring in the evaluation and management of undiagnosed chronic hip pain in a young adult. Physical Therapy 78(1): 62–73

POSTSCRIPT

Since the above article was written the author has undertaken a series of studies to explore some of the hypotheses presented. The result of most immediate interest was a study that demonstrated a change in the neuromuscular synergy of the hip abductors. It had been predicted that during a stepping task the stance limb of subjects with hip OA would demonstrate an increased activation of TFL and a decreased activation of GMed. This proposal was consistent with both clinical theory (Janda 1983; Sahrmann 2002) and experimental evidence (Long et al 1993). However, in the hip OA subjects there was an increased activation of the GMed and a nonsignificant trend toward increased TFL activation (Sims et al 2002).

Whilst there are several possible interpretations of this finding (see Sims et al 2002) the results provide support for the hypothesis presented in the above article highlighting the adverse effects of increased muscle forces. This proposal had been first suggested by Barrie (1986) as a possible explanation of wear patterns in the cartilage of subjects with hip OA. One possible explanation of these changes could be that altered afferent input from a diseased joint leads to an inefficient scaling of muscle forces appropriate to the task. Alternatively, pain may lead to a guarding action in the muscles around the joint. Experimental evidence suggests increased levels of gluteal muscle activity are associated with electrical stimulation of the pig sacroiliac joint (Indahl et al 1999).

These results have also directed the author's attention to the potential effects of increased levels of muscle activity on joint range of motion. Many of the muscles surrounding the hip have intimate capsular attachments, e.g. TFL, rectus femoris and pectineus (Williams et al 1995) and tonic activity in these muscles may, therefore, lead to capsular restriction. This is not a new concept. Muscle spasm leading to hip contracture was discussed many years ago (Pearson & Riddell 1962). The key in clinical practice is to identify factors contributing to overload in certain muscle groups. These include pain, habitual movement patterns and loss of normal muscular synergies. A well-known example of this latter point would be a dominance of the TFL over the GMed in a hip abduction synergy. A less discussed possibility is a dominance of the deep external rotators over the GMed and gluteus maximus in hip rotation leading to a loss of internal rotation.

The possibility that a change in the control of the centre of mass may have some relationship to the development of hip OA was also explored in the article above. Kinematic analysis of centre of mass motion in subjects with hip OA has not provided clear evidence for this hypothesis. This does not preclude the possibility but serves to reinforce the notion that hip OA has a multifactorial aetiology.

REFERENCES

Barrie HJ 1986 Unexpected sites of wear in the femoral head. Journal of Rheumatology 13(6): 1099–1104
Indahl AK, Kaigle A, Reikaras, O; Holm, S 1999 Sacroiliac joint involvement in activation of the porcine spinal and gluteal musculature. Journal of Spinal Disorders 12(4): 325–330
Janda V 1983 Muscle Function Testing. Butterworths, London & Boston
Long W, Dorr L, Healy B, Perry J 1993 Functional recovery of noncemented total hip arthroplasty. Clinical Orthopaedics and Related Research 288(March): 73–77

Pearson J, Riddell D 1962 Idiopathic osteoarthritis of the hip. Annals of Rheumatic Diseases 21: 31–39
Sahrmann S 2002 Diagnosis and Treatment of Movement Impairment Syndromes. Mosby, St Louis, USA
Sims K, Richardson C, Brauer S 2002 Investigation of hip abductor activation in subjects with clinical unilateral hip osteoarthritis. Annals of Rheumatic Diseases 61(8): 687–692
Williams P, Bannister L, Gray H 1995 In: Williams P (ed.) Gray's Anatomy. 38th edn. Churchill Livingstone, Edinburgh & New York

The Knee

SECTION CONTENTS

4

Management of patellofemoral problems

J. McConnell

McConnell and Clements Physiotherapy, Mosman, Sydney, Australia

Patellofemoral pain is often a challenge for the physiotherapist, because of its complex aetiology. Physiotherapists with their understanding of soft tissue structure and muscle function are well positioned to effectively manage most patello-femoral problems by improving the extensibility and mobility of tight structures and improving the timing of the elongated muscles. This will involve recognizing the biomechanical factors contributing to the symptoms, adequately explaining to the patient the cause of the symptoms and teaching the patient how to manage the symptoms. Specific training of certain muscles with accurate feedback to change the timing of these muscles during functional and sporting activities will be required if this problem is not to recur. *Manual Therapy*(1996) **1**, 60–66

INTRODUCTION

Patellofemoral pain is a common condition presenting to physiotherapists (Lutter 1985; Fulkerson & Hungerford 1990; Brukner & Khan 1993). The 25% of the population who will at some stage in their lives suffer from patellofemoral symptoms demonstrate a failure of the intricate balance of the soft-tissue structures, mostly due to inherent biomechanical faults (Radin 1979; Aglietti et al 1983; Hvid 1983; Grana & Kriegshauser 1985; Kramer 1986; Lyon et al 1988; Fulkerson & Hungerford 1990; Brukner & Khan 1993). This soft-tissue balance is particularly critical in the first 20° of knee flexion, where the position of the patella relative to the femur is determined by the interaction of the medial and lateral soft tissue structures. After the first 20° of knee flexion, as the patella engages in the trochlea, the bony architecture becomes increasingly responsible for the joint stability. Any imbalance in the soft-tissue structures in the first 20° of knee flexion will mean that the patella does not enter the trochlea optimally. This will cause undue stress on various tissues around the joint. The physiotherapist can influence the way the patella enters the trochlea by improving the flexibility of the passive structures, as well as improving the function of the active stabilizers of the joint.

The passive structures are more extensive and stronger on the lateral side than they are on the medial side, with most of the lateral retinaculum arising from the iliotibial band (ITB). If the ITB is tight, excessive lateral tracking and/or lateral patellar tilt can occur (Fiske-Warren & Marshall 1979; Dahhan et al 1981; Reider et al 1981; Fulkerson & Hungerford 1990). Active medio-lateral stabilization is provided by the quadriceps muscle, on the lateral side the vastus lateralis (VL) and on the medial side the vastus medialis (VM).

The fibres of the VL are orientated 12–15° laterally in the frontal plane. Vastus lateralis has an anatomically distinct group of distal fibres, the vastus lateralis oblique (VLO), which interdigitate with the lateral intermuscular septum before inserting into the patella (Hallisey et al 1987). The VLO fibres provide a direct lateral pull on the patella because of the interdigitation with the lateral intermuscular septum.

The vastus medialis is more distinctly divided than the VL, due to the orientation of its fibres. The fibres are divided functionally into two components — the longus, where the fibres are orientated 15–18 degrees medially to the frontal plane and the obliquus, where the fibres are orientated 50–55° medially in the frontal plane (Lieb & Perry 1968). The vastus medialis longus (VML) acts with the rest of the quadriceps to extend the knee. Although the vastus medialis obliquus (VMO) does not extend the knee, it is active throughout knee extension to keep the patella centred in the trochlea of the femur (Lieb & Perry 1968). The VMO arises from the tendon of the adductor magnus (Bose et al 1980) and is supplied in most cases by a separate branch of the femoral nerve (Lieb & Perry 1968).

The VMO is the only active medial stabilizer of the patellofemoral joint; therefore the timing and amount of activity in the VMO is critical to patellofemoral function. Small changes in this activity will have significant effects on the patellar position relative to the femur. A reduction in VMO tension of 50% results in a 5 mm displacement of the patella laterally (Ahmed et al 1988). A small effusion in the knee may contribute to the decrease in VMO tension, because VMO is inhibited when only 20 ml of fluid is present in the knee joint, whereas VL and rectus femoris are inhibited when an excess of 60 ml of fluid is present in the joint (Spencer et al 1984). The selective atrophy of the VMO with effusion may explain the increased incidence of patellofemoral symptoms following other knee trauma or pathology, where a small low-grade effusion seems to contribute to poor VMO activation.

VMO activation can be measured electromyographically, giving information about the intensity and timing of the muscle activity. Electromyographic (EMG) studies of normal subjects have revealed that the VMO:VL ratio should be 1:1, that the VMO has faster reflex response times compared with the VL and that the VMO displays tonic activity (Mariani & Caruso 1979; Reynolds et al 1983; Voight & Weider 1991). On the other hand, EMG recordings in patellofemoral pain sufferers have revealed that the ratio of VMO:VL is less than 1:1, the VL fires significantly faster than the VMO and the VMO demonstrates phasic activity (Mariani & Caruso 1979; Reynolds et al 1983; Voight & Weider 1991).

If the VMO is deactivated or the tension in the VL is twice that of the VMO, then the pressure distribution on the articular surfaces changes, such that it is concentrated on the lateral facet of the patella. Pressure on the lateral facet will, in turn, adversely affect the nutrition of the articular cartilage in the central and medial zones of the patella. Degenerative change will occur more readily in these areas. Therefore, one of the aims of management of patellofemoral problems is to facilitate a balance between the medial and lateral structures, so that the load through the joint is distributed as evenly as possible, particularly as the compressive force through the patellofemoral joint increases with increasing knee flexion. Other factors that may contribute to poor patellofemoral contact through abnormal patellofemoral mechanics include an increased Q angle, tightness in the lateral structures, faulty foot mechanics and poor timing of the gluteus medius and VMO muscles (Ahmed et al 1983; Fulkerson & Hungerford 1990; Brukner & Khan 1993). To adequately address the problems of faulty mechanics the physiotherapist must perform a thorough assessment.

CLINICAL EXAMINATION

The clinical examination establishes the neuro-musculoskeletal diagnosis and determines the underlying causative factors of the patient's symptoms so that the appropriate treatment can be implemented. In the history, the physiotherapist needs to establish the area of pain, the type of activity precipitating the pain, the history of the onset of the pain, the behaviour of the pain and any associated clicking, giving way or swelling (Brukner & Khan 1993). This gives an indication of the structure involved and the likely diagnosis; for example, if the type of activity that precipitated the patient's inferior patellar pain was one that involved eccentric loading, such as jumping in basketball or increased hill work during running, patellar tendonitis would be suspected (Brukner & Khan 1993; Molnar & Fox 1993). On the other hand, if the patient reported inferior patellar pain following tumble turning or vigorous kicking in the pool, an irritated fat pad would be suspected (McConnell 1991). This patient's pain would be aggravated by straight leg raise exercises, and hence it is essential the therapist recognizes the condition so that appropriate management can be implemented to enhance, rather than impede, recovery.

The patient with patellofemoral pain usually complains of a diffuse ache in the anterior knee which is exacerbated by stair climbing and prolonged sitting with the knee flexed — the movie sign (Cox 1985; Jacobson & Flandry 1989; Fulkerson & Hungerford 1990; Brukner & Khan 1993). Crepitus, giving way, locking and mild-swelling are other common symptoms but these symptoms must be differentiated from tibiofemoral intra-articular pathology. When considering the possible differential diagnoses, the physiotherapist must be aware that the lumbar spine and the hip can sometimes refer symptoms to the knee. For example, the prepubescent male with a slipped femoral epiphysis may present with a limp and anterior knee pain, and therefore can initially be misdiagnosed as having patellofemoral pain (Fulkerson & Hungerford 1990; Brukner & Khan 1993).

POSTURAL ANALYSIS

To determine the biomechanical asymmetries contributing to the patient's symptoms, the physiotherapist should initially examine the patient's limb alignment in standing. Biomechanical asymmetries such as internal femoral rotation (see Fig. 4.1), anterior or posterior pelvic tilt, hyperextended or 'locked back' knees, genu varum or valgum and abnormal pronation of the foot will affect the patient's gait pattern. For example, a patient with internally rotated femurs, posteriorly tilted pelvis and hyperextended knees will usually have poor inner-range quadriceps control and will not use knee flexion for shock absorption on heel strike, but will increase the amount of lateral pelvic tilt (trendelenberg appearance). Consequently, the lateral structures (ITB and lateral retinaculum) will lack flexibility and the gluteus medius muscle will lack control.

FUNCTIONAL ANALYSIS

The dynamic component of the assessment not only examines the effect of the static mechanics on the patient's movement, but aims to reproduce the patient's symptoms sothat the effect of the physiotherapeutic intervention can be determined. The least stressful activity of walking is examined first. If the patient's symptoms are not provoked in walking, then evaluation of more stressful activities such as stair climbing are performed. If symptoms are still not provoked then squat and one-leg squat may be examined and used as a re-assessment activity. Once a re-assessment activity has been obtained, the patient

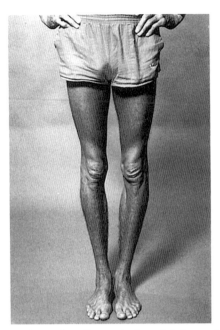

Figure 4.1 Lower leg alignment of a patellofemoral pain sufferer.

is evaluated in supine. With the patient in supine lying, the physiotherapist can exclude intra-articular pathology, can examine the passive movements of the knee, can test the hamstrings, iliopsoas, rectus femoris, tensor fascia latae, gastrocnemius and soleus muscles for length and can assess the position of the patella relative to the femur.

EXAMINATION OF PATELLAR POSITION

The physiotherapist needs to consider the patellar position, not with respect to the normal, but with respect to the optimal (McConnell 1986, 1987). An optimal patellar position is one where the patella is parallel to the femur in the frontal and the sagittal planes; and the patella is midway between the two condyles when the knee is flexed to 20° (McConnell 1986, 1987). The position of the patella is determined by examining four discrete components: glide, lateral tilt, anteroposterior tilt and rotation in a static and dynamic manner.

Determination of the glide component involves measuring the distance from the midpole of the patella to the medial and lateral femoral epicondyles. The patella should be sitting equidistant (±5 mm) from each epicondyle when the knee is flexed to 20°. In some instances, the patella may sit equidistant to the condyles, but moves laterally out of the line of the femur when the quadriceps contracts, indicating a dynamic problem. The dynamic glide examines both the effect of the quadriceps contraction on the patellar position, as well as the timing of the activity of the different heads of quadriceps. The VMO should be activated slightly earlier than VL (Voight & Weider 1991). In patients with patellofemoral pain the VMO activity is often delayed (Voight & Weider 1991).

If the passive lateral structures are too tight, then the patella will tilt laterally, such that the medial border of the patella will be higher than the lateral border and the posterior edge of the lateral border will be difficult to palpate. The lateral tilt, if severe, can lead to excessive lateral pressure syndrome (Fulkerson & Hungerford 1990). When the patella is moved in a medial direction, it should initially remain parallel to the femur. If the medial border of the patella rides anteriorly away from the femur, when the patella is pushed medially, the therapist can conclude that the patient has a dynamic lateral tilt problem. The patella, which, at full extension is sitting slightly lateral in the trochlea, should move medially to be centred in the trochlea as soon as the knee flexes. If the deep lateral retinacular structures are tight then the patella will not seat uniformly in the trochlea, so there will be an uneven distribution of load through the joint. If the lateral retinacular structures are tighter more distally on the patella, then the patella will externally rotate and if the tightness is greater at the superior pole, the patella will internally rotate. External rotation is a more common finding than internal rotation.

A rotation of the patella is determined by examining the position of the long axis of the patella relative to the long axis of the femur. Ideally, the long axis of the patella should be parallel to the long axis of the femur. If the inferior pole is sitting lateral to the long axis of the femur, the patient has an externally rotated patella. If the inferior pole is sitting medial to the long axis of the femur, then the patient has an internally rotated patella.

An optimal position also involves the patella being parallel to the femur in the sagittal plane. A most common finding is a posterior displacement of the inferior pole of the patella. This will result in fat pad irritation and often manifests itself as inferior patellar pain, which is exacerbated by extension manoeuvres of the knee (McConnell 1991). A dynamic posterior tilt problem occurs when the inferior pole of the patella is pulled posteriorly into the fat pad during a quadriceps contraction, particularly if the knee hyperextends.

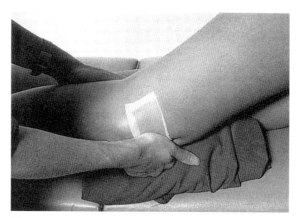

Figure 4.2 Therapist mobilizing the deep lateral retinacular structures.

TREATMENT

The aims of treatment for patellofemoral problems are to optimize the patellar position and toimprove the lower limb mechanics. An optimal patellar position is achieved by stretching the tight lateral structures and by changing the activation pattern of the VMO. Stretching the tight lateral structures can be facilitated passively, by both the therapist mobilizing the lateral retinaculum and the ITB (Fig. 4.2) and the patient, performing a self-stretch on the retinacular tissue (Fig. 4.3). However, the most effective stretch to the adaptively shortened retinacular tissue is obtained by a sustained low load, using, in this situation, tape to facilitate a permanent elongation of the tissues (Frankel & Nordin 1980; Hooley et al 1980; McKay-Lyons 1989; Taylor et al 1990; Herbert 1993).

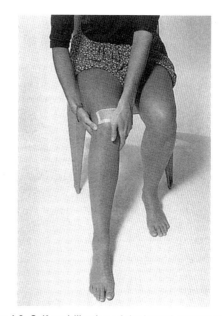

Figure 4.3 Self-mobilization of the lateral structures.

TAPING OF THE PATELLA — PASSIVE STRETCHING OF THE LATERAL RETINACULUM

The tape combination used on the patella is unique to each patient. It is determined by the assessment of the patellar position. The most abnormal component is usually corrected first, but

if a posterior tilt of the patella is present, the tape must be placed over the superior aspect of the patella, because taping more distally can aggravate the fat pad and exacerbate the patient's pain. The symptom-producing activity should be reassessed after each piece of tape is applied, to determine whether further correction is necessary. The tape should immediately improve a patient's symptoms by at least 50%. If the tape does not decrease the symptoms by 50%, then the therapist needs to consider whether:

1. The patient requires unloading tape, as well as the patellar tape
2. The tape was poorly applied
3. The assessment of patellar position was inadequate
4. The patient has an intra-articular primary pathology that is inappropriate for taping.

Correction of the glide component involves placing a piece of non stretch tape from the lateral patellar border and firmly pulling it to just past the medial femoral condyle. At the same time the soft tissue on the medial aspect of the knee is lifted towards the patella to create a tuck or fold in the skin superomedially. This provides a more effective correction of the glide component and also minimizes the friction rub (friction between the tape and the skin), which is relatively common in patients with extremely tight lateral structures. In many instances, hypoallergenic tape is placed underneath the rigid sports tape to provide a protective layer for the skin.

The lateral tilt component is corrected by firmly taping from the middle of the patella to the medial femoral condyle. The object is to lift the lateral border of the patella away from the femur, thereby stretching the deep lateral retinacular structures. Tight deep lateral retinacular structures is one of the commonest findings when assessing patellar position. Patellar rotations are corrected by taping from the poles of the patella to either turn the inferior pole upwards and medially (external rotation correction; see Fig. 4.4) or, less frequently, the superior pole downwards and medially (internal rotation correction).

Further taping to unload painful soft tissue structures may be required. The principle of unloading is based on the premise that inflamed soft tissue does not respond well to stretch. For example, if a patient presents with a sprained medial collateral ligament, applying a valgus stress to the knee will aggravate the condition, whereas a varus stress will decrease the symptoms. The same principle applies for patients with an inflamed fat pad, an irritated ITB or a pes anserinus bursitis. The inflamed tissue needs to be shortened or unloaded. To unload the fat pad, for example, the tape is applied to form a 'V' shape from the tibial tubercle to the medial and lateral joint lines. As the tape is being pulled towards the joint line, the skin is lifted towards the patella, thus shortening the fat pad (Fig. 4.5).

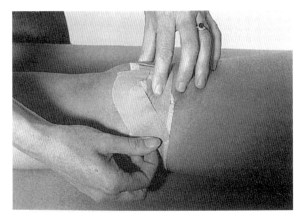

Figure 4.4 External rotation correction with tape.

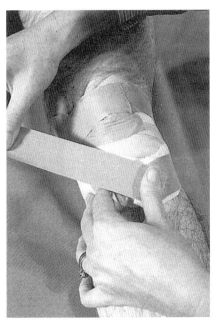

Figure 4.5 Unloading the fat pad.

The tape is kept on all day everyday until the patient has learnt how to activate the VMO at the right time; that is, the tape is like trainer wheels on a bicycle and can be discontinued once the skill is established. The patient should never train with or through pain or effusion (Spencer et al 1984; Stokes & Young 1984). If the patient experiences a return of the pain, then he or she should readjust the tape. If the activity is still painful, the patient must cease the activity immediately. The tape will loosen quickly if the lateral structures are extremely tight or the patient's job or sport requires extreme amounts of knee flexion.

VASTUS MEDIALIS OBLIQUUS TRAINING — ACTIVE STRETCHING OF THE LATERAL RETINACULUM

In the early stages of rehabilitation the emphasis should be given to the timing and intensity of the VMO contraction relative to the VL. The VMO should come in slightly earlier than the VL (Voight & Weider 1991). Biofeedback machines, particularly dual channel devices, are extremely useful to facilitate this process because they provide immediate feedback that reinforces the correct activation pattern (LeVeau & Rogers 1980; Wild et al 1982; Wise et al 1984; Ingersoll & Knight 1991). Weight-bearing activities need to be commenced early in rehabilitation to improve the muscle activation for functional activities. It has been proposed that training causes changes within the nervous system that allow an individual to better coordinate the activation of muscle groups (Sale 1987). For patients finding it difficult to change the VMO timing, the physiotherapist can emphasize adduction in the training, because it has been found that activation of the adductor magnus to 20% of its maximal will cause a differential increase in VMO activity relative to VL (Hodges & Richardson 1993). In non-weight bearing, however, a maximal contraction of the adductor magnus is required before any increase in activity in VMO relative to VL occurs (Hodges & Richardson 1993).

A useful starting exercise is small-range knee flexion and extension movements (the first 30° of knee flexion) with the feet apart. The weight is distributed either equally on both feet, or partially through the symptomatic limb. The VMO should be constantly active during this exercise, as it is in the first 20° where VMO recruitment is critical to the optimal seating of the patella in the trochlea. Figure 4.6 shows a patient performing small squats with the biofeedback electrodes placed on the VMO and the VL. The exercise can be progressed such that the patient is in a walk stance position. This position simulates the motion of the knee during the stance phase of walking. The patient should be relatively pain-free during all muscle training. If the patient's symptoms return, then the tape may have loosened during the course of treatment, and it should be readjusted so the patient can proceed with the training. For a patient who is having difficulty contracting the VMO, muscle stimulation may be used to facilitate the contraction.

As many patients experience pain during stair ascent and descent, another goal of treatment is to improve the patient's ability to negotiate stairs without reproducing symptoms. The patient

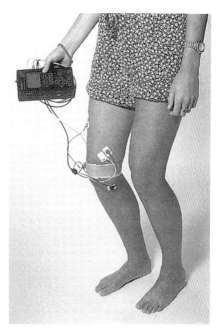

Figure 4.6 Dual channel biofeedback used to improve timing during small range squats.

needs to practise stepping down from a small height initially. This should be performed slowly, in front of a mirror, so that changes in limb alignment can be observed and deviations can be corrected. Specific work on the hip musculature may be necessary to improve the limb alignment. A stable pelvis will minimize unnecessary stress on the knee. Internal rotation of the hip increases the valgus vector force at the knee and can cause an increase in patellofemoral pain. If the anterior hip structures are flexible and the gluteals, particularly the posterior fibres of gluteus medius, are working well, there will be diminished activity in the tensor fascia lata (TFL). The decrease in activity in the TFL will result in a decreased lateral pull on the patella which, because the patella is not being displaced laterally, will enhance VMO activity (Ahmed et al 1988). It is usually necessary to remind the patient where the gluteus medius is, if specific training of the gluteus medius is required.

The number of repetitions a patient performs should be increased as the skill level improves because the VMO is a stabilizing muscl; therefore endurance training is the ultimate goal (Richardson & Bullock 1986). It is preferable for the therapist to emphasize quality not quantity. Initially, small numbers of exercises should be performed frequently throughout the day. The aim is to achieve a carry-over from functional exercises to functional activities. For further progression, the patient can move to a larger step, initially decreasing the number of contractions and slowly increasing them again. As the control improves, the patient can alter the speed of their stepping activity and may vary the place on descent where he/she stops going down. Weights may be introduced in the hands or in a backpa again the number of repetitions and the sp the movement should be decreased initia built back up again.

Training should be applicable to the pa activities/sport, so a jumping athlete example, should have jumping incorporat his/her programme. 'Figure of eight' run bounding, jumping off boxes, jumping ... turning and other plyometric routines particularly appropriate for the high-performa athlete. However, the VMO needs to be monitc at all times for timing and level of contracti relative to the VL. The number of repetitic performed by the patient at a training session w depend upon the onset of muscle fatigue. The ai would be to increase the number of repetitioi before the onset of fatigue. Patients should b taught to recognize muscle fatigue or quivering so that they do not train through the fatigue and risk exacerbating their symptoms.

The need for surgery for patellofemoral pain has almost been eliminated due to improved understanding of its aetiology, taping of the patella to reduce the symptoms and specific training of the VMO and gluteals. However, the patient needs to be aware that the symptoms are managed, not cured, and that the patellofemoral pain can recur, particularly when the activity level has increased and there has been a lapse in the exercise programme.

REFERENCES

Aglietti P, Insall J, Cerulli G 1983 Patellar pain and incongruence. Clinical Orthopaedics and Related Research 176: 217–224

Ahmed AM, Burke DL, Yu A 1983 In-vitro measurement of static pressure distribution in synovial joints—part II: Retropatellar surface. Journal of Biomedical Engineering 105: 226–236

Ahmed A, Shi S, Hyder A, Chan K 1988 The effect of quadriceps tension characteristics on the patellar tracking pattern. In: Transactions of the 34th Orthopaedic Research Society, Atlanta, p. 280

Bose K, Kanagasuntherum R, Osman M 1980 Vastus medialis oblique: an anatomical and physiologic study. Orthopaedics 3: 880–883

Brukner P, Khan K 1993 Clinical Sports Medicine. McGraw-Hill Co, Sydney, p. 316

Cox J 1985 Patellofemoral problems in runners. Clinics in Sports Medicine 4(4): 753–764

Dahhan P, Delphine G, Larde D 1981 The femoropatellar joint. Anatomica Clinica 3: 23–29

Fiske-Warren L, Marshall J 1979 The supporting structures and layers on the medial side of the knee. Journal of Bone and Joint Surgery 61A(1): 61

Frankel VH, Nordin M 1980 Basic Biomechanics of the Skeletal System. Lea and Febiger, Philadelphia

Fulkerson J, Hungerford D 1990 Disorders of the Patello-femoral Joint, 2nd edn. Williams & Wilkins, Baltimore

Grana WA, Kriegshauser LA 1985 Scientific basis of extensor mechanism disorders. Clinics in Sports Medicine 4(2): 247–257

Hallisey M, Doughty N, Bennett W, Fulkerson J 1987 Anatomy of the junction of the vastus lateralis tendon and the patella. Journal of Bone and Joint Surgery 69A(4): 545

Herbert R 1993 Preventing and treating stiff joints. In: Crosbie J, McConnell J (eds) Key Issues in Musculoskeletal Physiotherapy. Butterworth–Heinemann, Oxford, p. 114

P, Richardson CA 1993 An investigation into the tiveness of hip adduction in the optimisation of the us medialis oblique contraction. Scandinavian nal of Rehabilitation Medicine 25: 57–62

C, McCrum N, Cohen R 1980 The visco-elastic rmation of the tendon. Journal of Biomechanics 521

1983 The stability of the human patello-femoral joint. gineering in Medicine 12(2): 55

oll C, Knight K 1991 Patellar location changes llowing EMG biofeedback or progressive resistive xercises. Medicine and Science in Sports and Exercise 3(10): 1122–1127

bson K, Flandry F 1989 Diagnosis of anterior knee pain. Clinics in Sports Medicine 8(2): 179–195

mer PG 1986 Patella malalignment syndrome: rationale to reduce excessive lateral pressure. Journal of Orthopaedic and Sports Physical Therapy 8(6): 301–308

Veau B, Rogers C 1980 Selective training of the vastus medialis muscle using EMG biofeeback. Physical Therapy 60(11): 1410–1415

eb F, Perry J 1968 quadriceps function. Journal of Bone and Joint Surgery 50A(8): 1535–1548

utter L 1985 The knee and running. Clinics in Sports Medicine 4(4): 685–698

Lyon L, Benzl L, Johnson K, Ling A, Bryan J 1988 Q angle: a factor — peak torque occurrence in isokinetic knee extension. Journal of Orthopaedic and Sports Physical Therapy 9(7): 250–253

Mariani P, Caruso I 1979 An electromyographic investigation of subluxation of the patella. Journal of Bone and Joint Surgery 61: 169–171

McConnell J 1986 The management of chondromalacia patellae — a long term solution. Australian Journal of Physiotherapy 32(4): 215–223

McConnell J 1987 Training the vastus medialis oblique in the management of patellofemoral pain. In: Proceedings of Tenth Congress of the World Confederation for Physical Therapy, Sydney, May.

McConnell J 1991 Fat pad irritation — a mistaken patellar tendonitis. Sport Health 9(4): 7–9

McKay-Lyons M 1989 Low-load, prolonged stretch in treatment of elbow flexion contractures secondary to head trauma: a case report. Physical Therapy 69: 292

Molnar T, Fox J 1993 Overuse injuries of the knee in basketball. Clinics in Sports Medicine 12(2): 349–362

Radin E 1979 A rational approach to treatment of patellofemoral pain. Clinical Orthopaedics and Related Research 144: 107–109

Reider B, Marshall J, Koslin B, Ring B, Girgis F 1981 The anterior aspect of the knee. Journal of Bone and Joint Surgery 63A(3): 351–356

Reynolds L, Levin T, Medeiros J, Adler N, Hallum A 1983 EMG activity of the vastus medialis oblique and vastus lateralis in their role in patellar alignment. American Journal of Physical Medicine 62(2): 61–71

Richardson CA, Bullock MI 1986 Changes in muscle activity during fast alternating flexion and extension movements of the knee. Scandanavian Journal of Rehabilitation Medicine 18: 51–58

Sale D 1987 Influence of exercise and training on motor unit activation. Exercise and Sports Science Review 5: 95–151

Spencer J, Hayes K, Alexander I 1984 Knee joint effusion and quadriceps reflex inhibition in man. Archives of Physical Medecine 65: 171–177

Stokes M, Young A 1984 Investigations of quadriceps inhibition: Implications for clinical practice. Physiotherapy 70(11): 425–428

Taylor D, Dalton J, Seaber A 1990 Visco-elastic properties of muscle-tendon units. The biomechanical effect of stretching. American Journal of Sports Medecine 18: 300

Voight M, Weider D 1991 Comparative reflex response times of the vastus medialis and the vastus lateralis in normal subjects and subjects with extensor mechanism dysfunction. American Journal of Sports Medicine 10: 131–137

Wild J, Franklin T, Woods GW 1982 Patellar pain and quadriceps rehabilitation — an EMG study. American Journal of Sports Medicine 10(1): 12

Wise HH, Fiebert IM, Kates JL 1984 EMG feedback as a treatment for patellofemoral pain syndrome. Journal of Orthopaedic and Sports Physical Therapy 6(2): 95–103

POSTSCRIPT

There has been an increase in research investigating the management of patellofemoral pain in the last few years. Recently an extensive double-blind, randomized, placebo-controlled, multi-centre clinical trial conducted through The University of Melbourne has demonstrated that physiotherapy is successful in reducing pain and improving timing of the vastii during a stair-stepping task in patients with patellofemoral pain (Crossley et al 2002; Cowan et al 2002a). Seventy one patellofemoral pain syndrome patients were randomly allocated to a placebo or treatment group in one of ten private practices across Melbourne where they received six treatment sessions over 6 weeks. The treatment group received patellofemoral taping such that the symptoms were relieved by 50%, specific VMO training with biofeedback, hamstrings and anterior hip joint capsular stretches and gluteal training in a weight-bearing position. The placebo group received placebo taping along the line of the femur, detuned ultrasound and medicated gel. Blinding the subjects was highly successful, as 70% of the subjects in the placebo group thought were in the treatment group. Both groups reported an improvement in symptoms; however, individuals in the physiotherapy treatment group had significantly greater improvements than those in the placebo group in self-reported pain and disability scales, as well as in functional measures of stair stepping and squats. It was also identified that physiotherapy treatment changed the onset timing of the VMO relative to the VL during stair stepping and postural perturbation tasks. At baseline in both the placebo and treatment groups, the VMO came on significantly later than the VL. Following treatment, there was no change in muscle onset timing in the placebo group, but in the physiotherapy group, the onset of VMO and VL occurred simultaneously during concentric activity and the VMO actually preceded VL during eccentric activity, (Fig. 4.7) (Cowan et al 2002).

The control and timing of the muscles of the lower limb are critical to the smooth functioning

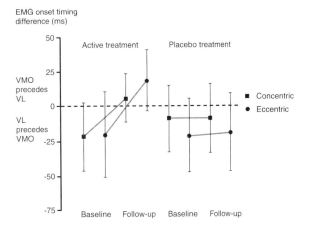

Figure 4.7 EMG changes following 6 weeks of physiotherapy treatment.

of the patellofemoral joint. However, the issue of quadriceps muscle imbalance and onset timing of the vastii in individuals with patellofemoral disorders is still controversial in the literature. Some investigators have found no difference in VMO and VL timing in PF sufferers, whereas others have found a delay in the onset of VMO relative to the VL (Voight & Weider 1991; Karst & Willett 1995, Witvrouw et al 1996; Powers et al 1997; Gilleard et al 1998; Sheehy et al 1998; Cowan et al 2002b). Some of the controversy may arise because there are too few subjects in some of these studies, potentially causing a type II error. In a recently completed study of 66 subjects with and without PF pain, Cowan and colleagues found that even though the majority of patellofemoral sufferers had a delayed onset of VMO relative to VL on a stair-stepping task (67% concentrically, 79% eccentrically), there were still some whose VMO preceded VL activation (Cowan et al 2001a). Thus, not all patients with PF pain have a VMO timing deficit — some may have a problem with the magnitude of the contraction or a coordination problem of the hip and knee musculature; others may have some other biomechanical abnormality contributing to their symptoms. Additionally, these investigators found that some of the asymptomatic subjects exhibited a delayed onset of the VMO relative to the VL (46% concentrically and 52% eccentrically) on the stair-stepping task (Cowan et al 2001b). Could these asymptomatic individuals be at risk for developing PF symptoms at some time in the future?

From the recent evidence it can be concluded that specific physiotherapy is successful in managing patellofemoral pain. If a therapist follows the programme outlined in this article, then the management of patellofemoral pain should no longer be a conundrum.

REFERENCES

Cowan SM, Bennell KL, Crossley KM, Hodges PW, McConnell J 2001a Physiotherapy treatment changes motor control of the vastii in patellofemoral pain syndrome (PFPS): A randomised, double-blind, placebo controlled trial. Medicine and Science in Sports and Exercise 33(5): S89

Cowan SM, Bennell KL, Hodges PW, Crossley KM, McConnell J 2001b Delayed onset of electromyographic activity of vastus medialis obliquus relative to vastus lateralis in subjects with patellofemoral pain syndrome. Archives of Physical Medicine and Rehabilitation 82(2): 183–189

Cowan SM, Bennell KL, Crossley KM, Hodges PW, McConnell J 2002a Physical therapy treatment alters recruitment of the vastii in patellofemoral pain syndrome. Medicine and Science in Sports and Exercise 34(12): 1879–85

Cowan SM, Hodges PW, Bennell KL, Crossley KM, McConnell J 2002b Altered vastii recruitment when people with patellofemoral pain syndrome complete a postural task. Archives of Physical Medicine and Rehabilitation 83(7): 989–95

Crossley K, Bennell K, Green S, Cowan S, McConnell J. 2002 Physical therapy for patellofemoral pain: A randomised, double-blind, placebo controlled trial. American Journal of Sports Medicine 30(6): 857–65

Gilleard W, McConnell J, Parsons D 1998 The effect of patellar taping on the onset of vastus medialis obliquus

and vastus lateralis muscle activity in persons with patellofemoral pain, Physical Therapy; 78(1): 25–32

Karst G, Willett G 1995 Onset timing of electromyographic activity in the vastus medialis oblique and vastus lateralis muscles in subjects with and without patellofemoral pain syndrome. Physical Therapy. 75(9): 813–822

Powers CM, Landel R, Sosnick T, Kirby J, Mengel K, Cheney A, Perry J 1997 The effects of patellar taping on stride characteristics and joint motion in subjects with patellofemoral pain Journal of Orthopaedic Sports Physical Therapy 26(6): 286–291

Sheehy P, Burdett RG, Irrgang JJ, Van Swearingen J 1998 An electro-myographic study of vastus medialis oblique and vastus lateralis activity while ascending and descending steps. Journal of Orthopaedic Sports Physical Therapy 27(6): 423–429

Voight M, Weider D 1991 Comparative reflex response times of the vastus medialis and the vastus lateralis in normal subjects and subjects with extensor mechanism dysfunction. American Journal of Sports Medicine 10: 131–137

Witvrouw E, Sneyers C, Lysens R, Jonck L, Victor J 1996 Comparative reflex response times of vastus medialis obliquus and vastus lateralis in normal subjects and subjects with patellofemoral pain syndrome. Journal of Orthopaedic Sports Physical Therapy 24(3): 160–166

SECTION 4

The Foot

SECTION CONTENTS

5

Achilles tendinopathy

J. L. Cook* K. M. Khan† C. Purdam‡
*Musculoskeletal Research Centre, La Trobe
University, Victoria, Australia
†Department of Family Practice (Allan McGavin
Sports Medicine Centre), School of Human Kinetics,
University of British Columbia, Canada
‡Head of Physiotherapy and Massage, Australian
Institute of Sport, Canberra, Australia

Achilles tendon injury (tendinopathy) and pain occur in active individuals when the tendon is subject to high or unusual load. Achilles tendinopathy can be resistant to treatment, and symptoms may persist despite both conservative and surgical intervention. The pathology of overuse tendinopathy is noninflammatory, with a degenerative or failed healing tendon response. The diagnosis of Achilles tendinopathy requires excellent differential diagnosis and an understanding of the role of tendon imaging. Conservative treatment must include exercise, with a bias to eccentric contractions. Surgical treatment is effective after complete tendon rupture, but may not assist recovery from overuse tendinopathy. Further research into the clinical aspects of Achilles tendinopathy is required. *Manual Therapy* (2002) **7(3)**, 121–130.

INTRODUCTION

Achilles tendon injury is a common sequel to sporting participation. Similar to the case with other tendons, pain classically appears with an increase in training load, or, in elite athletes, sustained high training loads. It appears more prevalent in sports that have a large running component, but occurs in all sports and at all levels of participation. Occasionally, Achilles tendon pain is found in inactive individuals.

Active older individuals may also present with Achilles tendon problems, often with symptoms for the first time. Occasionally, they can recall a previous episode or previous symptoms, or report asymptomatic tendon swelling for an extended period. Although age increases tendon cross-links and decreases tendon water content (Tuite et al 1997) and it may increase the degree of histopathological changes (Astrom & Rausing 1995), ageing is not specifically associated with tendinopathy (Maffulli et al 2000). Adolescent injury is uncommon, and childhood symptoms appear restricted to the region of the growth plate (Cameron et al 1994).

Injury is most commonly due to overuse, although acute complete ruptures also occur. Partial ruptures, although frequently diagnosed, may represent acute pain from pre-existing but asymptomatic tendinopathy, which may be evident on imaging (Gibbon et al 1999). Partial tears are frequently reported in surgical series in individuals with long-standing Achilles tendinosis (Astrom 1997). It remains unclear whether normal tendon with tightly bundled Type I collagen fibres can rupture in the transverse plane in small sections of a tendon. Pathology studies to date describe longitudinal separation and unplaiting of tendons rather than frank transverse tearing (Józsa et al 1990, 1991).

ANATOMY

The Achilles tendon is the single tendon of the soleus and gastrocnemius muscles, inserting into the calcaneum. It has a highly structured peritendinous tissue with no synovial membrane. The blood supply to the tendon enters on the deep (anterior) surface, and appears to be similar in volume throughout its length (Ahmed et al 1998). The presence of a hypovascular region that has been suggested to be a predisposing factor for midtendon tendinopathy was not supported in a study in which laser Doppler flowmetry (Astrom & Westlin 1994) was used.

The Achilles tendon lies close to several structures that are important in differential diagnosis of lower leg pain. These structures include the sural nerve, the posterior ankle structures, the medial tendons of the foot and toes and the bursae near the calcaneum. Pathology in these surrounding structures can mimic

Achilles tendon pain, either in the midtendon or insertional area.

MICROANATOMY

Normal tendon structure comprises sparse spindle-shaped tendon cells interspersed with a highly organized extracellular matrix. The tendon cells are responsible for the synthesis of all components of the extracellular matrix.

The matrix has tight bundles of long strands of Type I collagen, which give the tendon its inherent strength. Between the collagen, and a vital part of tendon structure, is the ground substance, made up of mainly small proteoglycans and glycosaminoglycan chains. In a normal tendon, there is minimal ground substance and it is not evident under light microscopic examination. Connective tissue (endotendon) lies parallel with the collagen bundles, enclosing and separating tendon fascicles (Fig. 5.1). Vascular and neural structures run between the collagen fascicles in conjunction with this connective tissue (O'Brien 1992).

The peritendon is a fine, loose connective tissue sheath comprising the epitenon (over the tendon) and the paratenon (outer layer). Connective tissue of the peritendon and the tendon are continuous with each other. The Achilles peritendon does not have a synovial layer found in hand and wrist tendons but is differentiated posteriorly into a number of fine gliding membranes lubricated by mucopolysaccharides (Lang 1960).

HISTOPATHOLOGY

Tendons respond poorly to overuse, and healing is slow, incomplete and lacks extracellular organization. This has been termed tendon degeneration (Leadbetter 1992), but may be more accurately defined as a failed healing response (Clancy 1989). This process leaves the pathological tendon substantially defective, which decreases tendon strength and leaves it less able to tolerate load and, thus, vulnerable to further injury.

Acute tendon injuries heal with a standard triphasic response, i.e. inflammation, proliferation

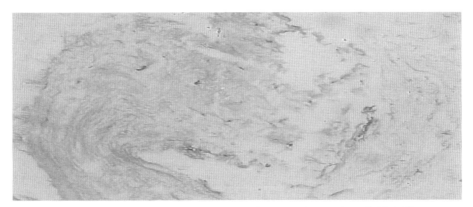

Figure 5.1 Light microscopic section of normal Achilles tendon (with permission Prof. N. Maffulli).

and maturation, and a structure that resembles normal tendon organization slowly re-forms (Frank et al 1999). It is unclear why overuse tendinopathy does not respond in this triphasic fashion. The process of tendon disruption that leads to micro-injury is unknown, and it may fail to stimulate an inflammatory response, adequate to begin the reparative cycle. Surgery for tendons that fail conservative treatment injures the tendon and creates a vascular disruption, which stimulates the triphasic repair process.

Microscopically, pathological tendon is in direct contrast to normal tendon, and the hallmarks of overuse tendinopathy are distinct. Primarily, large increases in the amount of ground substance are apparent, and this material has a greater proportion of large proteoglycans than found in normal tendon (Benazzo et al 1996).

Increases in ground substance are associated with disruption of the collagen bundles and their hierarchical arrangement (Astrom & Rausing 1995), and a decrease in amount of Type I collagen. Type III collagen is the collagen produced by the cells in response to injury; however, it is thinner and less able to bundle than Type I collagen.

There is an increase in the number of tendon cells, and immigration of fibroblasts from the peritendon, and perhaps other areas of tendon may be the source of these cells. The cells become active — rounded in appearance and have increased numbers of organelles responsible for protein synthesis (collagen and ground substance) (Fig. 5.2).

Some areas of tendinopathy become acellular (cystic tendinopathy) (Khan et al 1996) or have decreased cell numbers and function (hypoxic degeneration) (Józsa et al 1990). The cause of different cellular reactions and, consequently, different types of pathology, is unknown. Several types of pathology can be found in the same tendon.

Vascularity is increased in tendinopathy (Ohberg et al 2001); some new vessels are reported to be thick walled and tortuous, and have small lumina. The function of these vessels is questionable as the tendon surrounding them does not appear to have an advanced repair process (Kraushaar & Nirschl 1999).

The large amounts of ground substance, inferior collagen and vascularity are randomly arranged and lack organization, making the tendon less load tolerant. Exercise may offer a stimulant to improving the organization of these components (Wren et al 2000); however, further research is required. Peritendinous injury is a rarer presentation in the spectrum of Achilles tendon injury. Repeated cyclic movement of the tendon, such as cycling, may aggravate the peritendon. Peritendinopathy can exist by itself or in conjunction with tendinopathy (Khan et al 1999). In contrast to tendon injury, peritendinitis is distinctly inflammatory in nature (Kvist et al 1992).

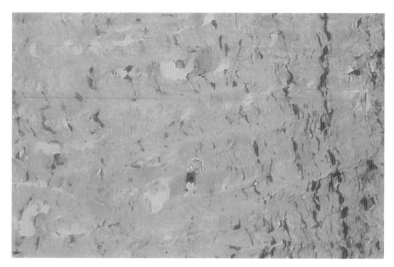

Figure 5.2 Achilles tendinopathy. Note the increase in cell population (with permission Prof. N. Maffulli).

AETIOLOGY OF ACHILLES TENDON INJURY

The Achilles tendon is reported to be affected by the biomechanics of the foot, the footwear of the person and the relative range of motion in the foot and ankle joint. Clinically, it is assumed that the behaviour of the foot in walking and running affects the homogeneity of the Achilles tendon load, but this is not supported in some research (Astrom 1997).

Research suggests that decreased ankle dorsiflexion is a risk factor for Achilles tendon pain (Kaufman et al 1999). This appears logical clinically, as the tendon must absorb load over a shorter range of movement and in less time.

Change in tendon load is also reported to be associated with Achilles tendon symptoms (Clement et al 1984), and clinically this is reported regularly. As yet, it has not been shown what amount of load or what change in load will increase tendon pathology or symptoms.

DIAGNOSIS

Achilles tendon injury is one of the simpler clinical diagnoses to make. The history is classic for both acute and overuse tendon injury and inflammation of the peritendinous tissues. In overuse tendinopathy, the person can often recall a change in activity levels or training techniques, with an insidious and gradual increase in symptoms. Originally the pain may not be disabling, but with continued activity, it can begin to affect the person's ability to train effectively. Rest will often relieve symptoms, but return to activity reactivates the pain, generally within a few training sessions.

The Achilles tendon is the only major tendon that must tolerate almost the full range of movement, including stretch, immediately on rising in the morning. Hence, morning pain is a hallmark of Achilles tendinopathy; the degree and time of stiffness are considered good indicators of tendon health and recovery from injury. Rest from training can also decrease morning stiffness, but often it will return with an increase in activity.

Symptoms of tendinopathy are localized to the tendon and immediate surrounding area. As tendon pain is usually localized to the tendon and does not appear to be referred to other regions, symptoms that are vague or encompass a larger area are suggestive of another source of pain, or perhaps tendon pain in conjunction with other pathology.

VISA-A Achilles tendon questionnaire

In this questionnaire, the term pain refers specifically to pain in the Achilles tendon region

1. For how many minutes do you suffer stiffness in the Achilles region on first getting up?

100 mins · | 1 2 3 4 5 6 7 8 9 10 | · 0 mins · POINTS ☐

2. Once you are warmed up for the day, do you have pain when stretching the Achilles tendon fully over the edge of a step (keeping knee straight)?

Strong severe pain · | 1 2 3 4 5 6 7 8 9 10 | · No pain · POINTS ☐

3. After walking on flat ground for 30 minutes, do you have pain for the next 2 hours?
(If unable to walk on flat ground for 30 minutes because of pain, score 0 for this question.)

Strong severe pain · | 1 2 3 4 5 6 7 8 9 10 | · No pain · POINTS ☐

4. Do you have pain walking downstairs with a normal gait cycle?

Strong severe pain · | 1 2 3 4 5 6 7 8 9 10 | · No pain · POINTS ☐

5. Do you have pain during or immediately after doing 10 (single leg) heel raises from a flat surface?

Strong severe pain · | 1 2 3 4 5 6 7 8 9 10 | · No pain · POINTS ☐

6. How many single leg hops can you do without pain?

None · | 1 2 3 4 5 6 7 8 9 10 | · No pain · POINTS ☐

7. Are you currently undertaking sport or other physical activity?

0 ☐ Not at all
4 ☐ Modified training ± modified competition
7 ☐ Full training ± competition, but not at the same level as when symptoms began
10 ☐ Competing at the same level or higher than when symptoms began

8. Please complete **EITHER A, B or C** in this question
- If you have **no pain while undertaking Achilles tendon loading sports** please complete **Q8A only**.
- If you have **pain while undertaking Achilles tendon loading sports but it does not stop you from completing the activity**, please complete **Q8B only**.
- If you have **pain which stops you from completing Achilles tendon loading sporting activities**, please complete **Q8C only**.

A. If you have no pain while undertaking Achilles tendon loading sport, for how long can you train/practise?

Nil	1–10 min	11–20 min	21–30 min	>30 min	POINTS
☐	☐	☐	☐	☐	☐
0	7	14	21	30	

OR

B. If you have some pain while undertaking Achilles tendon loading sport, but it does not stop you from completing your training/practice, for how long can you train/practise?

Nil	1–10 min	11–20 min	21–30 min	>30 min	POINTS
☐	☐	☐	☐	☐	☐
0	4	10	14	20	

OR

C. If you have pain that stops you from completing your training/practice in Achilles tendon loading sport, for how long can you train/practise?

Nil	1–10 min	11–20 min	21–30 min	>30 min	POINTS
☐	☐	☐	☐	☐	☐
0	2	5	7	10	

TOTAL SCORE (/100) ☐ %

Figure 5.3 VISA-A Achilles tendon questionnaire.

The VISA-A (see Fig. 5.3) scale is a subjective rating scale that quantifies the symptoms and dysfunction in the Achilles tendon (Robinson et al 2001). This assessment tool is very useful to rate Achilles tendons and to assess progress of recovery during rehabilitation. Other clinical tests and questionnaires have also been used to evaluate treatment outcomes (Silbernagel et al 2001).

Acute tendon rupture will be reported as a sensation of a blow on the tendon and a loss of function, but may not be associated with considerable pain. Peritendinitis results in crepitus, swelling and exquisite tenderness.

On examination, the tendon can appear completely normal, but more often will have subtle changes in outline, becoming thicker in both the anteroposterior and mediolateral plane. The increase in anteroposterior diameter may be difficult to detect clinically, but is classically in the midtendon, and can be very focal or broader in area.

Swelling and pain at the attachment is less common and must be assessed fully differential diagnosis includes pain associated with bony prominences (Haglund's deformity, pump bumps, calcaneal spurs) and bursae (Haglunds, retrocalcaneal). Longitudinal and transverse tears at the bone–tendon junction have been demonstrated at this site (Rufai et al 1995). Athletically, pain at the insertion may be seen in individuals with large range of dorsiflexion where the calcaneum can impinge on the anterior aspect of the tendon. Insertional pain may have a systemic cause and this aetiology must be fully explored.

A complete examination of the athlete should include the biomechanics of the foot, ankle and leg during walking and running, and include slow-motion analysis. Barefoot and examination in athletic shoes and with and without orthotics (if used) should be carried out. Range of ankle dorsiflexion should be quantified in standing and the difference between the neutral foot and the pronated foot used should be noted. The number and quality of single leg heel raises and hops, noting pain and endurance, should be recorded.

Finally, gentle palpation of the tendon and surrounding structures and the calf muscle should be carried out. Palpation tenderness may guide the examiner to the area of tendon that has subtle swelling or specific nodules. Palpation should include assessment of tendon compliance, muscle tightness, and fluctuance of swelling (Williams 1986).

Palpation tenderness is not a clinically useful diagnostic sign as small amounts of pressure provoke pain in tendons. Palpation tenderness has been shown not to correlate with imaging changes or symptoms in the patellar tendon (Cook et al 2001).

Peritendon involvement can be difficult to assess clinically, although full blown peritendinitis is easily recognized, with exuberant swelling, crepitus and the classic sign of the swelling not moving with tendon movement. More commonly, the line between tendon-only and combined pathology can only be assessed effectively by imaging.

A complete rupture can be determined from the calf squeeze test (Maffulli 1998); squeezing the calf in prone does not elicit any movement of the foot. Partial ruptures are impossible to diagnose clinically and present an imaging dilemma as well, as long-standing tendinopathy may appear on imaging with discontinuity of collagen fascicles.

IMAGING

Superficial tendons are very amenable to imaging with ultrasound and the Achilles is no exception. Ultrasound images provide a clear indication of tendon width, changes of water content within the tendon and peritendon and collagen integrity. A normal tendon appears consistent in width and anteroposterior diameter with continuous fascicles and thin hyperechogenic peritendinous structures (Fig. 5.4).

In contrast, an abnormal tendon will reveal at the very least an increase in tendon diameter, but often shows areas of increased water (hypoechochenicity), collagen discontinuity and tendon sheath swelling. Small areas of calcification may also be visible.

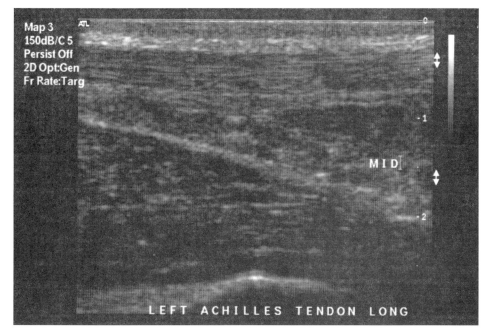

Figure 5.4 A normal Achilles tendon.

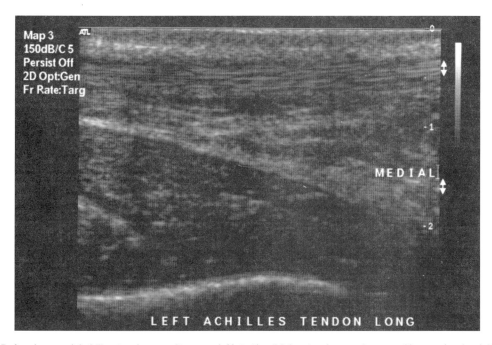

Figure 5.5 An abnormal Achilles tendon on ultrasound. Note the thicker tendon, and areas of hypoechochenicity.

Ultrasound can also detect bursal swelling, an important differential diagnosis in Achilles tendinopathy (Gibbon et al 2000) (Fig. 5.5).

Ultrasound should be the imaging modality of first choice in Achilles tendon, as it is inexpensive and readily available, and clearly defines the pathology (Davies et al 1991). If the diagnosis is unclear or the symptoms are atypical, magnetic resonance imaging (MRI) may be worth while. MRI is also very sensitive to pathology, which appears as increased signal within the Achilles tendon (Haims et al 2000) (Fig. 5.6). MRI is often most effective when several structures in the region need imaging.

DIFFERENTIAL DIAGNOSIS

A multitude of structures are implicated in the differential diagnosis in the Achilles region but a good clinical examination should allow accurate diagnosis. Posterior ankle impingement, medial tendon tendinopathy, and bursitis are relatively easy to diagnose. Sural nerve symptoms and referred pain from a spinal region are more difficult to diagnose.

Pain that is nonspecific in nature and not clearly related to tendon loading is clue to these more complex diagnoses which, should include systemic inflammatory diseases. Sciatic nerve

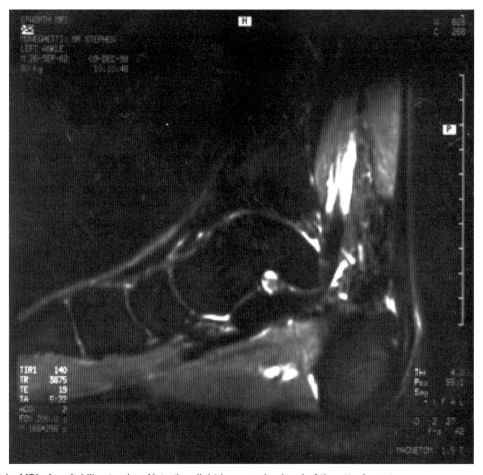

Figure 5.6 An MRI of an Achilles tendon. Note the slight increase in signal of the attachment.

irritation may be associated with Achilles tendon rupture through several possible mechanisms (Maffulli et al 1998).

TREATMENT OF TENDINOPATHY

The object of any treatment in any condition is to decrease pain and improve tissue function. In tendinopathy the source of the pain is undefined (Khan & Cook 2000), and the effect of conservative or physiotherapeutic interventions on tendinopathic tissue is poorly understood. We are therefore forced to acknowledge that whilst some interventions have been demonstrated to improve musculotendinous function, we are currently unable to define how, where and why this occurs.

Musculotendinous strengthening seems to be essential in tendon rehabilitation. It appears that the nature of this strengthening programme should be strongly biased towards eccentric muscle contraction (Mafi et al 2001). It is unclear if eccentric muscle contraction equips the muscle for better sporting function, or if it directly affects tendon pathology, as the stimulus for repair in pathologic tendon tissue remains elusive. It should be considered, however, that exercise appears to be the only stimulus described to date that positively influences collagen alignment (Kannus et al 1997).

Rest as a treatment for tendinopathy stems from the previous inflammatory paradigm of tendinitis, and will be effective in reducing pain, but offers no improvement in musculotendinous function. In fact rest appears to affect tendon tissue negatively, reducing collagen amount and strength (Kannus et al 1997).

CONSERVATIVE TREATMENT

As exercise-based programme is essential in tendon rehabilitation, appropriate and progressive exercises must be prescribed if rehabilitation is to succeed. Inadequate amounts of load, speed and endurance may result in incomplete rehabilitation and insufficient musculotendinous strength to return to sport.

Eccentric exercise was first reported by Curwin and Stanish (1984) as a useful intervention for tendinopathy. They reported that eccentric exercise resolved symptoms in a 6-week period. The programme was progressed by increasing speed and load, subject to symptoms. A recent study by Alfredson et al (1998) reported excellent results with heavy load eccentric exercise. This programme varied considerably from that proposed by Curwin and Stanish in that speed was not used as a progression of the exercise, pain was not a contraindication to continuing exercises and the eccentric component of the exercise was completed single leg.

Currently, this regime remains the gold standard for Achilles tendon rehabilitation and appears effective in most athletes. Recent studies have further supported the use of eccentric exercise (Silbernagel et al 2001). In competitive athletes, the exercise programme may need to be progressed to a level beyond that prescribed by Alfredson, in order to address specific muscle hypertrophy, speed, strength and endurance requirements in specific sports.

Manipulation of training load in athletes may be an essential management strategy in conjunction with an eccentric exercise programme. Reduction of volume, intensity, speed and repetitions may all spare the tendon sufficiently to reduce symptoms and allow progression of rehabilitation. Occasionally, complete rest or cessation of training may be required to settle severe symptoms.

Electrophysical modalities are useful to modulate pain and appear to be more effective in well vascularized tissue. As tendon pain commonly produces symptoms under load, and is poorly vascularized, these modalities offer little in the treatment of Achilles tendinopathy.

The effectiveness of manual therapy for the Achilles tendon remains unclear. In vitro studies suggest that physical manipulation of tendon cells may affect the cellular output (Almekinders et al 1993); however, there is little evidence that this occurs in vivo (Wilson et al 2000). Hunter (2000) proposes tendon mobilization and restoration of accessory movement of the tendon and surrounding structures. Massage for pertendinitis will increase the inflammatory reaction and is not recommended.

Ensuring flexibility of the musculotendinous unit and the ankle joint is an important component of rehabilitation. In some athletes effective ankle joint interventions may be difficult, as many jumping sports are associated with recurrent ankle injury, talocrural degeneration and anterior impingement. Improving ankle dorsiflexion in any athlete is difficult, and only small gains may be possible. Flexibility of both components of the calf is important, and stretches should address this. Regular massage during rehabilitation is beneficial to assist muscle recovery during the strengthening process. Specific soft tissue releases may also be utilized.

Correction of biomechanical imperfections is clinically important even if it is unclear if this directly affects tendon recovery. Alteration in the amount and/or speed of foot pronation is considered to be the most useful intervention. Control of foot mechanics in athletes is best achieved with tailored, rigid orthotic prescription. Heel raises to decrease tendon load are also often prescribed but the effectiveness of this has not been demonstrated.

Long-term follow-up (mean 8 years) of Achilles tendon patients has shown that one third required surgery, but of those that responded to a variety of conservative management, most recovered fully (Paavola et al 2000).

DIFFICULT TENDONS

When pain prevents an athlete training and playing, full attention and compliance to rehabilitation is possible. However, when an athlete can continue to train or compete with pain, rehabilitation becomes more complex. Introducing exercises to strengthen the musculotendinous unit appears unnecessary, as maximal muscle function should be gained during training. Despite athletic competence and ability to remain competitive, athletes often favour their symptomatic leg and place excessive load onto the unaffected leg, resulting in loss of strength and function, despite ongoing sports participation.

Hence, specific exercise programmes tailored to these deficits may still have a place in the competing athlete.

Poor compliance to load management and exercise by athletes decreases the effectiveness of rehabilitation. These athletes may partially recover and return to abusive loads prematurely, only to have a return of pain. Several relapses will often force longer-term compliance on athletes; however some seek an 'easy' surgical treatment without understanding the implications of, and recovery time from, this intervention.

Some tendons fail to recover despite adequate practitioner and athlete involvement. Increased intensity of exercise (speed, change of direction), and return to training and competition are common points of failure. Further management may allow return to sport, but long-term training modification (training quality or quantity) may be necessary.

PERITENDINOUS TREATMENT

Acute peritendinopathy has been difficult to manage, with anti-inflammatory treatment offering somewhat mixed outcomes. More recently, and based on early work by Rais (1961), the use of heparin and its derivatives either locally within the peritendon or systemically has offered excellent clinical recovery in a few days. Chronic peritendinopathy will not respond to this regime.

SURGICAL TREATMENT

Failure to respond to a complete conservative rehabilitation programme necessitates surgical intervention if the athlete is to have an opportunity to return to sport at their desired level. Tendon surgery, however, does not guarantee success, and rehabilitation times are often prolonged and outcomes may be less than satisfactory (Maffulli et al 1999a). A recent review of Achilles tendon surgery by Tallon et al (2001) revealed experimental design flaws in some studies reporting outcomes after Achilles tendon surgery. Further high-quality research in this area is required.

TENDON RUPTURE

The Achilles tendon is the most common tendon to rupture spontaneously (Kannus & Józsa 1991). The highest incidence of tendon rupture occurs in men between 30 and 39 years, whereas women appear to be protected until the post-menopausal years (Maffulli et al 1999b). Tendons that rupture are nearly always pathological prior to rupture, although only one-third were reported to be symptomatic prior to rupture (Kannus & Józsa 1991).

Surgical repair after rupture is encouraged in those seeking to continue sports participation, as the re-rupture rate in those treated conservatively has been shown to be significantly higher than in those treated surgically (Moller et al 2001). If the tendon remains intact, the long-term outcome in those managed conservatively has been reported to be similar to those treated operatively (Bressel 2001); however, long-term deficits in endurance capacity, range of movement and calf bulk have also been reported (Horstmann et al 2000).

CONCLUSION

Achilles tendon injury is a relatively simple diagnostic condition in both acute and overuse injury. Recent techniques of rehabilitation produce a very good outcome in the majority of cases; however, the evidence that underpins the mechanism of effective treatment is lacking. Failure to respond to conservative treatment requires surgical treatment, although a satisfactory outcome following this procedure is not guaranteed. Further research is required to improve the management of this condition.

REFERENCES

Ahmed I, Lagoloulos M, McConnell P, Soames R, Sefton G 1998 Blood supply of the Achilles tendon. Journal of Orthopaedic Research 16(5): 591–596

Alfredson H, Pietila T, Jonsson P, Lorentzon R 1998 Heavy-load eccentric calf muscle training for the treatment of chronic Achilles tendinosis. American Journal of Sports Medicine 26(3): 360–366

Almekinders LC, Banes AJ, Ballenger CA 1993 Effects of repetitive motion on human fibroblasts. Medicine and Science in Sports and Exercise 25(5): 603–607

Astrom M 1997 On the nature and etiology of chronic Achilles Tendinopathy. Lund University, Sweden

Astrom M, Westlin N 1994 Blood flow in the normal Achilles tendon assessed by laser Doppler flowmetry. Journal of Orthopaedic Research 12(2): 246–252

Astrom M, Rausing A 1995 Chronic Achilles tendinopathy. A survey of surgical and histopathologic findings. Clinical Orthopaedics 316: 151–164

Benazzo F, Stennardo G, Valli M 1996 Achilles and patellar tendinopathies in athletes: pathogenesis and surgical treatment. Bulletin of the Hospital of Joint Disease 54: 236–240

Bressel E 2001 Biomechanical behavior of the plantar flexor muscle-tendon unit after an Achilles tendon rupture. American Journal of Sports Medicine 29(3): 321–326

Cameron DM, Bohannon RW, Owen SV 1994 Influence of hip position on measurements of the straight leg raise test. Journal of Orthopaedic and Sports Physical Therapy 19(3): 168–172

Clancy W 1989 Failed healing responses. In: Leadbetter W, Buckwater J, Gordon S (eds) Sports-Induced Inflammation: Clinical and Basic Science Concepts. American Orthopedic Society for Sports Medicine, Park Ridge, Il

Clement DB, Taunton JE, Smart GW 1984 Achilles tendinitis and peritendinitis. Etiology and treatment. The American Journal of Sports Medicine 12: 179–184

Cook J, Khan K, Kiss S, Purdam C, Griffiths L 2001 Reproducibility and clinical utility of tendon palpation to detect patellar tendinopathy in young basketball players. British Journal of Sports Medicine 35: 65–69

Curwin S, Stanish WD 1984 Tendinitis: its Etiology and Treatment. Collamore Press, Lexington

Davies SG, Baudovin CJ, King JB, Perry JD 1991 Ultrasound, computed tomography and magnetic resonance imaging in patellar tendinitis. Clinics in Radiology 43: 52–56

Frank C, Shrive N, Hiraoka H, Nakamura N, Kaneda Y, Hart D 1999 Optimisation of the biology of soft tissue repair. Journal of Science and Medicine in Sport 2(3): 190–210

Gibbon WW, Cooper JR, Radcliffe JS 1999 Sonographic incidence of tendon microtears in athletes with chronic Achilles tendinosis. British Journal of Sports Medicine 33:129–130

Gibbon W, Cooper J, Radcliffe G 2000 Distribution of sonographically detected tendon abnormalities in patients with a clinical diagnosis of chronic Achilles tendinosis. Journal of Clinical Ultrasound 28: 61–66

Haims A, Schweitzer M, Patel R, Hecht P, Wapner K 2000 MR imaging of the Achilles tendon: overlap of findings in symptomatic and asymptomatic individuals. Skeletal Radiology 29: 640–645

Horstmann T, Lukas C, Mayer F et al 2000 Isokinetic strength and strength endurance of the lower limb musculature ten years after achilles tendon repair. Isokinetics and Exercise Science 8: 141–145

Hunter G 2000 The conservative management of Achilles tendinopathy. Physical Therapy in Sport 1: 6–14

Józsa L, Kannus P, Balint JB, Reffy A 1991 Three-dimensional ultrastructure of human tendons. Acta Anatomica 142: 306–312

Józsa L, Reffy A, Kannus P, Demel S, Elek E 1990 Pathological alterations in human tendons. Archives of Orthopaedic and Trauma Surgery 110: 15–21

Kannus P, Józsa L 1991 Histopathological changes preceding spontaneous rupture of a tendon. Journal of Bone and Joint Surgery 73A: 1507–1525

Kannus P, Józsa L, Natri A, Jarvinen M 1997 Effects of training, immobilization and remobilization on tendons. Scandinavian Journal of Medicine and Science in Sports 7: 67–71

Kaufman K, Brodine S, Shaffer R, Johnson C, Cullison T 1999 The effect of foot structure and range of motion on musculoskeletal overuse injuries. American Journal of Sports Medicine 27(5): 585–593

Khan K, Cook J 2000 Overuse tendon injuries: where does the pain come from? Sports Medicine and Arthroscopy Reviews 8: 17–31

Khan KM, Bonar F, Desmond PM et al 1996 Patellar tendinosis (jumper's knee): findings at histopathologic examination, US and MR imaging. Radiology 200: 821–827

Khan KM, Bonar SF, Cook JL, Harcourt PR, Astrom M 1999 Histopathology of common overuse tendon conditions: update and implications for clinical management. Sports Medicine 6: 393–408

Kraushaar B, Nirschl R 1999 Tendinosis of the elbow (tennis elbow). Clinical features and findings of histological, immunohistochemical, and electron microscopy studies. Journal of Bone and Joint Surgery America 81(2): 259–278

Kvist M, Józsa L, Jarvinen M 1992 Vascular changes in the ruptured Achilles tendon and its paratenon. International Orthopaedics 16: 377–382

Lang J 1960 Gliding tissue of muscles, fascias and blood vessels. Zeitschrift fur Anatomie und Entwicklungsgeschichte 122: 197–231

Leadbetter W 1992 Cell matrix response in tendon injury. Clinics in Sports Medicine 11(3): 533–578

Maffulli N 1998 The clinical diagnosis of subcutaneous tear of the Achilles tendon. A prospective study in 174 patients. American Journal of Sports Medicine 26(2): 266–270

Maffulli N, Irwin A, Kenward M, Smith F, Porter R 1998 Achilles tendon rupture and sciatica: a possible correlation. British Journal of Sports Medicine 32: 174–177

Maffulli N, Binfield P, Moore D, King J 1999a Surgical decompression of chronic central core lesions of the Achilles tendon. American Journal of Sports Medicine 27(6): 747–752

Maffulli N, Waterston W, Squair J, Reaper J, Douglas H 1999b Changing incidence of Achilles tendon rupture in Scotland: a 15 year study. Clinical Journal of Sports Medicine 9(3): 157–160

Maffulli N, Barrass V, Ewen S 2000 Light microscopic histology of Achilles tendon ruptures. American Journal of Sports Medicine 28(6): 857–863

Mafi N, Lorentzon R, Alfredson H 2001 Superior short-term results with eccentric calf muscle training compared to concentric training in a randomized prospective multicenter study on patients with chronic Achilles tendinosis. Knee Surgery, Sports Traumatology, Arthroscopy 9: 42–47

Moller M, Movin T, Granhed H, Lind K, Faxen E, Karlsson J 2001 Acute rupture of the tendon Achilles. Journal of Bone and Joint Surgery 83B: 843–848

O'Brien M 1992 Functional anatomy and physiology of tendons. Clinics in Sports Medicine 11(3): 505–520

Ohberg L, Lorentzon R, Alfredson H 2001 Novascularisation in Achilles tendons with painful tendinosis but not in normal tendons: an ultrasonographic investigation. Knee Surgery, Sports Traumatology, Arthroscopy 9: 233–238

Paavola M, Kannus P, Paakkala T, Pasanen M, Jarvinen M 2000 Long-term prognosis of patients with Achilles tendinopathy. American Journal of Sports Medicine 28(5): 634–642

Rais O 1961 Heparin Treatment of peritenomyosis (peritendinitis) crepitans acuta. Acta Chirurgica Scandinavica Supplementum 268

Robinson JM, Cook JL, Purdam C et al 2001 The VISA-A questionnaire: a valid and reliable index of the clinical severity of Achilles tendinopathy. British Journal of Sports Medicine 35: 335–341

Rufai A, Ralphs JR, Benjamin M 1995 Structure and histopathology of the insertional region of the human Achilles tendon. Journal of Orthopaedic Research 13: 585–593

Silbernagel K, Thomee R, Thomee P, Karlsson J 2001 Eccentric overload training for patients with chronic Achilles tendon pain—a randomised testing of the evaluation methods. Scandinavian Journal of Medicine and Science in Sports 11(4): 197–206

Tallon C, Coleman B, Khan K, Maffulli N 2001 Outcome of surgery for chronic Achilles tendinopathy. American Journal of Sports Medicine 29(3): 315–320

Tuite DJ, Renstrom PAFH, O'Brien M 1997 The aging tendon. Scandinavian Journal of Medicine and Science in Sports 7: 72–77

Williams JG 1986 Achilles tendon lesions in sport. Sports Medicine 3: 114–135

Wilson JK, Sevier TL, Helfst R, Honong E, Thomann A 2000 Comparison of rehabilitation methods in the treatment of patellar tendinitis. Journal of Sports Rehabilitation 9: 304–314

Wren T, Beaupre G, Carter D 2000 Tendon and ligament adaptation to exercise, immobilisation and remobilisation. Journal of Rehabilitation Research and Development 37(2): 217–224

POSTSCRIPT

CONSERVATIVE TREATMENT

Recent investigations by Alfredson and colleagues have furthered the understanding of tendon pain. After demonstrating an increased volume of vascularity in painful tendons compared to normal tendons (Ohberg et al 2001), Ohberg and Alfredson 2002 have investigated the effect of closing these vessels by injecting a sclerosant under ultrasound control in a group of subjects with resistant symptoms (Ohberg & Alfredson 2002). In this treatment group, eight of the 10 subjects became pain-free after several injections (2–5 injections) directed at the increased vascularity. Follow-up ultrasound demonstrated a decrease in vessel numbers in the painfree subjects compared with those with continued symptoms.

This study suggests that increased vascularity or adjacent structures (nerves, lymph vessels) may be associated with tendon pain. Neural structures are associated with vascular structures in tendons. The sclerosant has been shown to affect the vessels, but it is possible that it also affects the adjacent nerves.

The authors suggest caution in interpreting this pilot work and further research is underway. The function of the vascularity in tendinopathy is questionable, although theorized to be necessary for repair, and the patency of the vessels has been questioned. They are reported to have small lumina, and to have a tortuous course, and are not to be associated with improved repair (Kraushaar & Nirschl 1999). However, it is clear from this and other studies (Astrom & Westlin 1994) that significant blood flow occurs in these vessels.

Although there is no evidence as yet that sclerosing them will compromise repair in the long term, this needs to be demonstrated in controlled trials. Similarly, if vessel reduction reduced pain in active athletes who induce high loads in the Achilles tendon, reduced pain perception may lead these athletes to load tendon to levels not tolerated in a painful tendon. The risk of any increased load in tendons with pathology and compromised vascularity needs to be fully assessed before such treatment options are offered to athletes.

The role of electrophysical agents in treatment of tendinopathy remains poorly investigated; however, a recent paper compared the outcome after hyperthermia with low-frequency microwave and traditional ultrasound in a randomized trial (Giombini et al 2002). Significantly better outcomes were recorded by the hyperthermia group immediately after treatment and 1 month later.

SURGICAL TREATMENT

A prospective study of surgery for overuse Achilles tendinopathy has shown that the outcomes after surgery are better for those tendons without a focal lesion compared with those with a focal area of tendinopathy (Paavola et al 2002). Although the follow-up in this study is short term (7 months), 67% had returned to physical activity — 88% in the no-lesion group and 50% in the group with a focal lesion. The activities each group participated in are not reported, so it is unclear if the activity levels were a factor in lesion development or recovery from surgery.

REFERENCES

Åstrom M, Westlin N 1994 Blood flow in Chronic Achilles Tendinopathy. Clinical Orthopaedics 308: 166–172

Giombini A, Cesare AD, Casciello G, Sorrenti D, Dragoni S, Gabriele P 2002 Hyperthermia at 434 MHz in the treatment of overuse sport tendinopathies: A randomised controlled clinical trial. International Journal of Sports Medicine 23: 207–211

Kraushaar B, Nirschl R 1999 Tendinosis of the elbow (tennis elbow). Clinical features and findings of histological, immunohistochemical, and electron microscopy studies. Journal of Bone and Joint Surgery 81A(2): 259–278

Ohberg L, Lorentzon R, Alfredson H 2001 Neovascularisation in Achilles tendons with painful tendinosis but not in normal tendons: an ultrasonographic investigation. Knee Surgery, Sports Traumatology, Arthroscopy 9: 233–238

Ohberg L, Alfredson H 2002 Ultrasound guided sclerosis of neovessels in painful chronic Achilles tendinosis: pilot study of a new treatment. British Journal of Sports Medicine 36: 173–177

Paavola M, Kannus P, Orava S, Pasanen M, Jarvinen M 2002 Surgical treatment for chronic Achilles tendinopathy: a prospective seven month follow up study. British Journal of Sports Medicine 36(3): 178–182

6

Static biomechanical evaluation of the foot and lower limb: the podiatrist's perspective*

L. M. G. Lang R. G. Volpe J. Wernick
Sheffield Hallam University, Sheffield UK; New York
College of Podiatric Medicine, New York, USA
* A collaborative paper between the Department of
Podiatry, University of Brighton, Eastbourne, UK and
the New York College of Podiatric Medicine, New
York, USA. (L. M. G. Lang previously worked at the
Univerity of Brighton, UK.)

A biomechanical assessment is one aspect of podiatry. It involves two main modes of examination: dynamic and static. Aspects of the static mode are described with particular emphasis on the foot. The static mode includes both open and closed kinetic chain examinations. Each part of the lower extremity is evaluated with reference to the planes of the body. In open-chain examination specific techniques have been developed to evaluate the quality and range of motion of the foot joints. The foot is held in a standardized position that simulates the midstance period of the gait cycle. The position and function of the subtalar joint is considered to be particularly influential in the foot. For this reason the method of manipulating the patient's subtalar joint into the 'neutral position' is important. In closed-chain examination, posture is evaluated in both 'relaxed' and 'neutral' stance positions. Dynamic and static biomechanical examination data have to be interpreted with reference to the primary complaint and a full medical history, together with specific information concerning footwear and the habitual loco-motor functional needs of the patient. *Manual Therapy* (1997) **2(2)**, 58–66

INTRODUCTION

In the health-care team, the work of the podiatrist is focused on the lower limb and, in particular, the foot. The integrity and mobility of the foot are essential for all forms of gait and stance. Disorders encountered include not only those arising locally within the foot; they may be local manifestations of much wider systemic diseases, such as diabetes.

An important and common group of disorders in podiatric practice involve the locomotor system. Faulty foot mechanics, for example, poor shock absorption due to subtalar and midtarsal joint dysfunction, may have repercussions presenting much more proximally, as for example in the spine causing low back pain (Minkowsky & Minkowsky 1996). Equally, extrinsic factors can play a dominant role in influencing foot function.

Often a brief clinical review of the patient's active and passive movements, static and nd dynamic function, is sufficient and forms part of the initial diagnostic evaluation. A full biomechanical assessment is obviously indicated when the history and presenting signs and symptoms point to locomotor dysfunction.

PRINCIPLES GOVERNING CLINICAL BIOMECHANICS

The basic principles of physics are fundamental to all biomechanical evaluations and the practitioner must understand and apply these principles (Root et al 1977; Rogers & Cavanagh 1986).

A thorough understanding of the gait cycle and functional demands made on joints and muscles during walking and running is essential to the podiatrist, together with a detailed knowledge of the functional anatomy. Each position, movement or abnormality is assessed with reference to the three planes of the body (Green & Carol 1984), for example the cardinal sagittal plane (midline of the body) is the reference plane for all transverse positions, movements or abnormalities.

The practitioner must know the range of normality and in particular be able to recognize where normality ceases and pathology begins.

Root et al (1971) proposed certain 'criteria of normalcy' and these are used by podiatrists to evaluate the foot and leg.

When the body attempts to overcome abnormal function at one point in the locomotor system it usually does so at the nearest point in the system where it can achieve the same or similar function. This is referred to as compensation. There are certain theorems of compensation that have been developed in podiatry to explain and predict biomechanical pathologies (pathomechanics) (Southerland & Orien 1995). In general, the joints of the foot, especially the subtalar and the midtarsal joints, are often primary sites of compensation. The subtalar joint is regarded as acting as the key between the leg and distal joint function in the foot (Close & Inman 1953). To perform this role the subtalar joint converts limb rotation into pronation and supination of the foot and is structurally and mechanically linked to the ankle and midtarsal joints (Elftman 1960; Bojsen-Moller 1979; Lang 1987; Lundberg et al 1989).

There must be an appreciation of the significance of evidence in biomechanical evaluation. The human body frequently is not symmetrical and yet symmetry is generally regarded as an important basis for normal bipedal walking and running. Podiatrists use a number of methods and measurements in evaluating the lower limb that are usually quite simple, but their clinical interpretation is often more complex. For example, an individual's tolerance to limb length asymmetry can depend on many more factors than the measured magnitude of the discrepancy (Beekman et al 1985). Indeed, measurement of the human body is not without error (Lang 1990; Blake & Ferguson 1992; Baggett & Young 1993). Thus, the experienced podiatrist recognizes that biomechanical evaluation is not only a science, but an art. Clinical experience and skill should provide the basis for the practitioner's decisions as to what is significant biomechanically and what is needed in the best interests of the patient.

Sound biomechanical evaluation involves two modes of examination: dynamic and static, the latter being in both open and closed kinetic chain. Convergent evidence from both of these sources contributes to the accuracy of the diagnosis. Each mode of evaluation requires special skills and merits more than one article. Biomechanical evaluation is a very wide subject with many shades of opinion. For these reasons this article will present the authors' personal experience and will mainly focus on the static mode of assessment, with particular emphasis on the foot. The following summarizes some of the concepts that the authors consider to be important in podiatric biomechanics:

- Subtalar joint function influences the range of motion of distal joints
- Primary compensation will take place in the nearest joint whose largest component of movement is in the same plane as that affected by pathology.
- The severity of resulting pathology is directly related to the time in the gait cycle when the primary joint compensates.
- The level of compensation will depend on the range of motion at the primary compensation site and the degree of abnormality.
- Severity will also be affected by weight, occupation, footwear and extrinsic influences, such as abnormalities located more proximally in the lower limb.

MAKING A CLINICAL BIOMECHANICAL ASSESSMENT

A full and comprehensive history is important. Age, weight, occupation, hobbies, sports and environment, especially the local environment of the foot, may all be relevant factors. Examination of the patient's everyday and sports footwear can provide valuable evidence concerning types of footwear used, the mechanics of the feet and how the patient habitually stands and walks with shoes (Fuller 1994).

The assessment begins as soon as the patient enters the consulting room. The way the patient walks, stands and sits can be very revealing and may usefully be compared with more formal assessments of gait analysis and standing posture, which may be made later in the consultation.

It is good practice to standardize the method and order of conducting a biomechanical assessment. While the dynamic examination will not be covered in depth in this article, the authors wish to stress its importance. It is recommended that, wherever possible, dynamic examination precedes static examination. Gait observations often direct the emphasis of the static evaluation. If, for example, a patient is seen to intoe in the dynamic examination, this would direct the static examination toward transverse plane factors, including hip rotation, knee position, malleolar angle and forefoot alignment, to rule out femoral anteversion, shortened muscle and ligaments, internal tibial torsion and metatarsus or forefoot adductus. On the other hand, in the case of a patient exhibiting a high 'bouncing' gait with an early heel rise, the static examination would focus on sagittal plane components to rule out ankle equinus and, if present, determine its origin and treatment.

Where necessary, video records may aid dynamic assessment. These provide a visual record and allow the practitioner to review the data. In certain cases, additional information concerning mechanical forces may be indicated. A number of podiatrists use barefoot or inshoe force or pressure measuring instrumentation to evaluate these parameters of gait (West 1987; Fuller 1996).

During the dynamic examination the practitioner may initially observe static stance. However, it is useful to undertake a more thorough evaluation of closed kinetic chain in stance after the 'open chain' examination. This enables the examiner to compare open and closed chain position and morphology. Further-more, any reference lines drawn with the patient recumbent can then also be used in the stance examination.

OPEN KINETIC CHAIN EXAMINATION

The extent of this part of the examination will vary according to the patient's history, presenting signs and symptoms and, of course, the findings of the gait analysis. In this account, examination of the limb proximal to the ankle will be covered briefly with the primary focus on evaluation of the foot.

In the open chain examination the flexibility of the joints and soft tissues in the lower limbs are assessed together with muscle strength. Both limbs are compared in their entirety, followed by the various segments, including their alignment. Any asymmetry is noted and, where necessary, length and circumference measurements are recorded.

HIP JOINT

Motion in all three body planes is compared on both sides and to the accepted normal ranges (Gastwirth 1996). Transverse plane range of movement is tested with hips flexed and extended. Restricted medial or lateral rotation that persists irrespective of hip flexion and extension is likely to be of bony origin and may require further investigation; if it is only observed with hips flexed or extended it is likely to be of soft tissue origin (Valmassey 1996). The power and flexibility of the iliopsoas and hamstring muscles may be assessed.

KNEE JOINT

Any evidence of joint disturbance is noted. The competence of the principal ligaments is tested and also the strength and flexibility of the quadriceps and hamstrings (Baylis & Rzonca 1988).

FOOT

The morphology of the non-weight-bearing foot is observed, particularly the appearance of the arches. The location and type of any mechanically induced skin or nail lesions are useful data concerning foot function.

ANKLE JOINT

The dominant plane of motion is sagittal around a single axis, which lies close to the frontal and transverse planes. However, as the axis crosses from the fibular to tibial malleolus it angles slightly to the other two planes and, therefore, gives triplane motion (Inman 1976; Lundberg et al 1989). In open chain examination the ankle joint is assessed by movement of the foot on the leg, but in walking when the foot is flat on the ground it is the leg that moves over the static foot (Perry 1992). It is generally accepted that about 10° of dorsiflexion is needed in midstance during barefoot walking (Root et al 1977; Lindsjo et al 1985). In the open chain examination the angle made by the foot to the lower leg is noted using the fibula as a guide or a bisection line on the lateral aspect of the leg and the contour of the lateral border of the foot (or heel in the case of forefoot equinus). This is done with the knee flexed and extended, with the subtalar joint in its neutral position to minimize the effects of pronation or supination, which can influence the apparent range of sagittal plane motion (Fig. 6.1). Diminished dorsiflexion with the knee extended compared with flexed suggests gastrocnemius tightness or passive insufficiency. Any general limitation of movement noted when compared with the other side may be due to osseous or articular abnormality and will require further investigation.

Malleolar angle may be assessed as an indicator of tibial or, more correctly, tibiofibular torsion. This is particularly indicated if intoeing is noted in the dynamic assessment or if the history of the complaint is consistent with compensation for an intoe problem, which more commonly presents in children. With the patient sitting, the knee is positioned by the examiner so that the femoral and tibial condyles are parallel to the examination couch. The ankle and subtalar joint positions are standardized in their neutral positions before the malleolar angle is assessed. Measurement can be made with reference to the horizontal supporting surface of the couch, using a goniometer aligned to the centres of the tibial and fibular malleoli (Valmassey 1996). Although it is generally accepted that, with the exception of neonates, the angle should be external, there is some dispute concerning normal values (Lang 1990). Means from as low as 13° to over 30° externally have been cited. As with all meas-

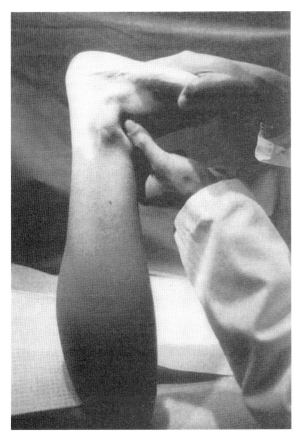

Figure 6.1 Ankle joint dorsiflexion tested with the subtalar joint in the neutral position.

urements the angle must be considered within the context of the overall clinical picture. However, an internal angle should be regarded as an abnormal finding at any age.

SUBTALAR JOINT

The subtalar joint is regarded as the key between the lower limb and the foot. The contour of the articular facets between the talus and calcaneum and the triplane axis (42° from the transverse plane, 16° from sagittal) enable this joint to convert transverse plane movements of the hip into pronation and supination in the foot (Manter 1941; Root et al 1966). The planar dominance of component movements differs with differences in axis angulation and foot morphology (Close

& Inman 1953; Root et al 1966). Furthermore, the subtalar joint influences joints distal to it, especially the midtarsal joint with which it is intimately structurally and functionally linked. Thus, it is important that this joint's position is standardized when distal joints are examined. Conventionally, the subtalar joint neutral position, defined as the point of maximum congruity when the joint is neither pronated or supinated, is used. It is located at the highest point of the arc of subtalar joint rotation and is assumed to be transected during walking in midstance (Wright et al 1964). Range and quality of motion are assessed with the patient lying prone. Because the frontal plane components of subtalar joint movement are more accessible than the movements in the other two planes, observation and evaluation is made of calcaneal inversion and eversion, with reference to the lower part of the leg. The examiner moves the foot through its range of motion by holding either the calcaneum or the fourth or fifth rays. The thumb and the index finger of the other hand palpate the medial and lateral surfaces of the subtalar joint just distal to the malleoli. When the joint is supinated the talus is prominent on the lateral aspect. In pronation it is prominent medially. To assist examination, and, where required, goniometric measurement, bisection lines may be drawn on the posterior surface of the lower one-third of the leg and calcaneum. When drawing these lines, it is important that the leg and heel posterior surfaces are in the frontal plane and that the examiner is looking directly over the part. The bisection of the leg should be over the soleus, between the distal end of the gastrocnemius and end above the tendocalcaneus. In the posterior heel the line should bisect the bony surface of the calcaneum and end above the subcutaneous fat pad of the heel (Fig. 6.2). The joint allows more supination than pronation. Root et al (1977) suggest a ratio of about 2:1, with an average total range of 30° of motion. Others suggest greater variability associated with differences in axis alignment (Close & Inman 1953; Wernick & Volpe 1996).

MIDTARSAL JOINT

The midtarsal joint a functional concept that involves two joints. The joint is also mechanically complex with two triplane axes of motion (Bojsen-Moller 1979). The oblique axis is so called because of alignment particularly to the sagittal and transverse planes of the body, giving supination with marked plantar flexion and adduction and pronation with marked dorsiflexion and abduction. The longitudinal axis gives greater frontal plane motion (Manter 1941; Root et al 1971, 1977; Wernick & Volpe 1996).

The midtarsal joint provides movement between the rear and forefoot. It facilitates shock absorption and maintains plantigrade foot posture in the presence of uneven terrain and changes in subtalar joint position (Phillips & Phillips 1983; Wernick & Volpe 1996). It directly influences the apparent heights of the medial and lateral longitudinal arches of the foot (Elftman 1960). Its mechanics appear to be unique to the human foot (Bojsen-Moller 1979).

In open chain assessment the midtarsal joint range and quality of motion around each of the axes are more easily assessed with the patient supine. It is important when testing the range of motion around each axis that the examiner stabilizes the ankle and subtalar joints in neutral positions with one hand, using the other hand to

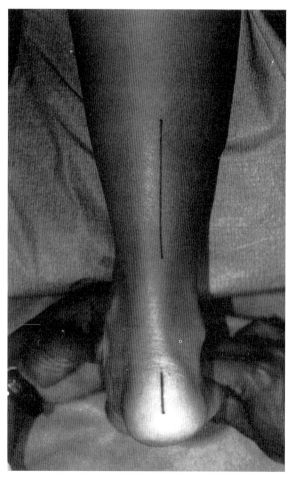

Figure 6.2 Open chain assessment of the subtalar joint: 'neutral position'.

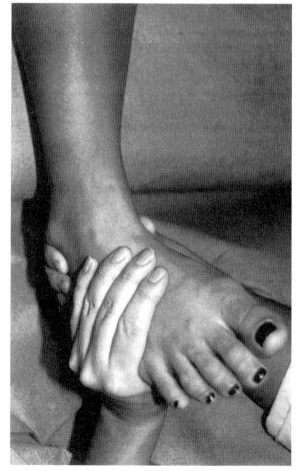

Figure 6.3 Midtarsal joint range of motion examination: oblique axis supination.

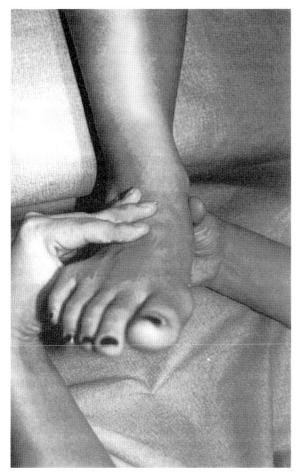

Figure 6.4 Midtarsal joint range of motion examination: oblique axis pronation.

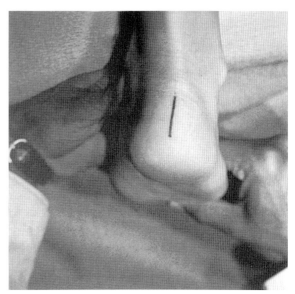

Figure 6.5 Forefoot to rearfoot alignment with subtalar joint in neutral and midtarsal joint pronated to resistance by loading fourth and fifth metatarsals distally.

foot, specifically with reference to the second to fourth metatarsal heads, should lie parallel to the plantar surface of the calcaneum and, therefore, at 90° to a bisection line on the posterior surface over the calcaneum (Fig. 6.5). If the forefoot were found to be inverted or everted with reference to the rearfoot, this would be considered to be an abnormal finding and could be either soft tissue or bony, i.e. forefoot varus or valgus.

THE RAYS OF THE FOREFOOT

The first and fifth rays are regarded separately as they each have their own axis, whereas the intermediate rays are believed to be much more stable and function as a unit (Root et al 1977). Whilst the axes of the first and fifth rays have yet to be precisely defined, they are considered to be triplane. However, the axis of the first ray differs in direction from other triplane axes in the foot since it crosses from medial to lateral, posterior to anterior and slightly plantarwards. Hence, this axis permits plantarflexion with some eversion and possibly slight abduction of the first ray and dorsiflexion with inversion and slight adduction (Root et al 1977; Weed & Root 1982). The fifth ray

rotate the midtarsal joint around each of its axes (Figs 6.3 & 6.4).

In standing and during the midstance period of the stance phase of the gait cycle the foot is plantigrade. The plantar aspects of fore- and rearfoot should be parallel to each other and to the supporting surface with the subtalar joint in neutral and the midtarsal joint pronated around its oblique axis. This is tested in open kinetic chain with the patient prone, the subtalar joint in its neutral position and the midtarsal joint pronated by manually loading the fourth and fifth metatarsal heads until the examiner feels the forefoot passively resist further movement. In this position the fore-

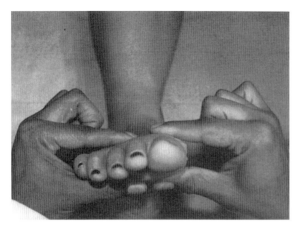

Figure 6.6 Examination of first ray position and motion.

consists of the fifth metatarsal and moves in supination and pronation.

Clinical evaluation is aimed at determining the relative position and range of dorsiflexion and plantarflexion of the first and fifth rays with reference to the more stable intermediate three rays. Specifically the first ray is compared to the second. Using the thumbs and index fingers the examiner holds the heads of the first and second metatarsals. With the subtalar joint in neutral the examiner dorsiflexes and plantarflexes the first ray to the point where the examiner feels passive resistance in each direction. Equal amounts of dorsiflexion and plantarflexion are considered to be normal, with the metatarsal head parallel to its neighbour in the resting position (Fig. 6.6). The fifth ray is evaluated in the same manner. The motion and position of the rays are clinically important in that they influence the mechanics of their associated metatarsophalangeal joint. This is particularly significant in the first ray because plantarflexion of the ray facilitates dorsiflexion of the first metatarsophalangeal joint during the propulsive phase of gait (Gudas 1979; Phillips et al 1996; Roukis et al 1996).

METATARSOPHALANGEAL JOINTS

These biaxial joints can each move independently around a transverse axis in dorsi- and plantarflexion and around a vertical axis in add- and abduction. The first joint is the most significant mechanically and in barefoot walking should be free to move to about 50° of dorsiflexion during the propulsive period of gait (Hetherington et al 1990). Limitation in this movement during walking has been cited as a cause of more proximal functional disturbance and certain related pathologies, such as excessively pronated feet, calcaneal spurs, arthritis of the knee joint and low back pain (Dananberg 1986, 1993). The quality and range of motion is evaluated with the subtalar joint in its neutral position and the examiner holding the proximal phalanx. A digital goniometer may be used to make any measurements required. However, it should be recognized that there is a distinction between functional dorsiflexion (in gait) and assisted dorsiflexion (in static examination) when higher values have been reported (Hetherington et al 1990).

STATIC CLOSED CHAIN EXAMINATION

The patient is observed in standing. Overall posture and segmental orientation is evaluated in each body plane. The patient may be first asked to walk 'on the spot' to simulate their angle and base of gait and their usual stance position (Fig. 6.7).

EXAMINATION OF THE FRONTAL PLANE (ANTERIOR ASPECT)

To put the patient at ease it is usually better to start with them facing the examiner. The examiner is positioned so as to be in line with the midline of the patient and able to observe alignment and symmetry in the frontal plane starting with the head, neck and shoulders. With the arms dependent the relative height of the finger tips can also be used to check shoulder tilt. A tilt to one side may be indicative of a structural or functional asymmetry and should be further investigated.

Next, the alignment of the pelvis and hips are checked, using the iliac crests for reference. This is followed by noting the angular alignment of the thighs and legs. The presence of genu valgum or varum is noted and, where indicated, the Q angle may be measured and/or the distance between the femoral medical condyles and tibial malleoli. Whilst checking the knees it is useful to use the patella as a landmark for transverse plane orientation of the thigh, noting whether it is central, or externally or internally orientated. Internal orientation may be associated with femoral anteversion or medial limb rotation. In the ankle, the relative height of the malleoli can be observed. A discrepancy at this level indicates asymmetrical pronation or supination. The position of the subtalar joints can be estimated by comparing the symmetry of the curves above and below the malleoli. Excessive pronation is suggested by a deeper concavity under the lateral malleolus relative to the supramalleolar curve often with a reduced or convex curve under the medial malleolus (Root et al 1971). Finally the feet are examined. The angle of the feet whether straight, abducted or adducted with reference to the midline of the body is noted. The position of the toes is noted together with any deformities.

EXAMINATION OF THE FRONTAL PLANE (POSTERIOR VIEW)

The basic features previously noted are checked again from a posterior view. Additional information includes direct observation of the spine if shoulders or pelvic tilt is apparent, also symmetry of the gluteal folds and flexure lines of the knee joints. The angle of the feet is reviewed and distance between the heels is used as an indication of the base of stance (Fig. 6.7).

Observation of the calcaneum will reveal the frontal plane alignment of the rear foot. The relaxed stance position, 'relaxed calcaneal stance', of the heel is noted, whether vertical, inverted or everted with reference to the ground. This is used as an indication of the frontal plane component of subtalar joint closed kinetic chain motion (in closed kinetic chain the calcaneum moves primarily in the frontal plane while the talus moves mainly in the transverse and sagittal planes). If required, measurement may be made with a protractor placed parallel to the heel on the

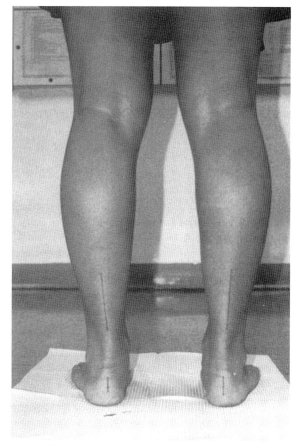

Figure 6.7 Relaxed calcaneal stance position with patient standing in their simulated angle and base of gait.

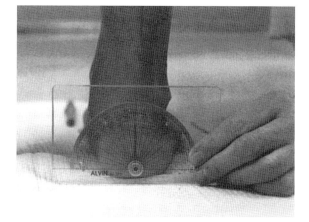

Figure 6.8 Measurement of subtalar joint to supporting surface alignment in closed kinetic chain examination: patient in relaxed calcaneal stance position.

supporting surface, the angle of the rear foot being measured using the previously drawn bisection line on the heel (Fig. 6.8). Also relevant to this is the related position of 'neutral calcaneal stance' in which the patient stands with the subtalar joint in its neutral position. A difference between these two values indicates the amount of compensation that has occurred at the subtalar joint. Various techniques can be used to achieve this position, including palpating the subtalar joint whilst rotating the leg until the neutral position is located (Figs 6.9 & 6.10) and observation of the alignment of the malleoli and the alignment of the leg over the foot (Root et al 1971, 1977; Cook et al 1988).

According to the 'criteria of normalcy' the leg and calcaneum should be vertical to the supporting surface (Root et al 1971). The leg may be assessed with reference to the line bisecting the lower one-third of the leg. This is checked both in relaxed and neutral calcaneal stance to discriminate between 'apparent' and 'true' bony angulation.

The contours of the medial and lateral borders of the foot are noted both in relaxed and subtalar neutral stances. In relaxed stance a convex medial and concave lateral border ('cuboid notch'), with apparent abduction of the forefoot with reference to the adducted rear foot, suggests midtarsal joint oblique axis pronation (Hice 1984). If so, the foot contours will usually straighten when the subtalar joint is moved into its neutral position.

EXAMINATION OF THE SAGITTAL PLANE

The patient should be observed from both sides. The angle of the head and neck is checked. Any deviation from the normal curvatures of the spine forward or backward is noted. In the lower limb the position of each joint is checked to determine if there is excessive flexion or extension.

In the foot the morphology of the longitudinal arches is considered from the medial and lateral aspects and compared with open kinetic chain appearance. A marked lowering of the arch in standing may indicate pronation, but soft-tissue

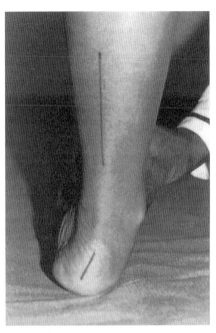

Figure 6.9 Examiner manipulating the subtalar joint through its range of motion in closed kinetic chain: supination.

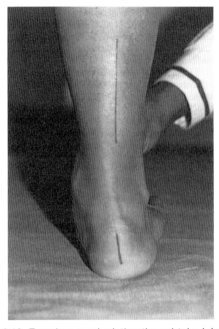

Figure 6.10 Examiner manipulating the subtalar joint through its range of motion in closed kinetic chain: pronation.

flexibility or limb position could be implicated (Muller et al 1993). While standing additional examination may include the great toe extension test. Assuming a mobile hallux, in a flexible flat foot, passive extension of the hallux will elevate the longitudinal arch, usually with associated external rotation of the leg (Rose et al 1985). Failure of this test to raise the arch indicates abnormal foot mechanics (Jack 1953; Rose et al 1985; Tachdjan 1985).

CONCLUSION

As in any branch of medicine, the final diagnosis and effective treatment can only be achieved by putting together and evaluating all the available evidence. This includes the patient's symptoms, history, footwear, the results of both dynamic and static modes of clinical biomechanical assessment, together with any additional specialized investigations such as force measurement. Whilst recognition of any abnormal function, e.g. excessive subtalar pronation in stance may be an important finding, it is not a diagnosis. Diagnosis requires establishing what is causing a manifest mechanical abnormality and relating it to the presenting complaint. It must be emphasized that the various components of a comprehensive biomechanical assessment should not be used in isolation, but rather be considered as a whole.

Acknowledgements

The authors wish to acknowledge the help of colleagues in the New York College of Podiatric Medicine (NYCPM) and University of Brighton. In particular staff of the NYCPM Library and the department of Information Services. We wish to thank Karl Petion, photographer, and third year students Joyce Feliciano, Camille Rodriguez and Patrick Sapini for help with illustrations.

REFERENCES

Baggett BD, Young G 1993 Ankle joint dorsiflexion. Journal of the American Podiatric Medical Association 83(5): 251–254

Baylis WJ, Rzonca EC 1988 Common sports injuries to the knee. Clinics in Podiatric Medicine and Surgery 5(3): 591–612

Beekman S, Louis H, Rosich JM, Coppola N 1985 A preliminary study on asymmetrical forces at the foot to ground interface. Journal of the American Podiatric Medical Association 75(7): 349–354

Blake RL, Ferguson H 1992 Limb length discrepancies. Journal of the American Podiatric Medical Association 82(1): 33–38

Bojsen-Moller F 1979 Calcaneo cuboid joint and stability of the longitudinal arch of the foot at high and low gear push off. Journal of Anatomy 129: 165–176

Close JR, Inman VT 1953 The action of the subtalar joint. Prosthetic Devices Research Project. Institute of Engineering Research, University of California Berkley 11(24)

Cook A, Gorman I, Morris J 1988 Evaluation of neutral position of the subtalar joint. Journal of the American Podiatric Medical Association 78(9): 449–451

Dananberg HJ 1986 Functional hallux limitus and its relationship to gait efficiency. Journal of the American Podiatric Medical Association 76(11): 648–652

Dananberg HJ 1993 Gait style as an etiology to chronic postural pain. Journal of the American Podiatric Medical Association 83(8): 433–441

Elftman H 1960 The transverse tarsal joint and its control. Clinical Orthopaedics 16(41): 41–45

Fuller EA 1994 A review of the biomechanics of shoes. Clinics in Podiatric Medicine 11(2): 241–258

Fuller EA 1996 Computerized gait evaluation. In: Valmassey RL (Ed). Clinical Biomechanics of the Lower Limb. Mosby Yearbook, St Louis, pp 179–206

Gastwirth BW 1996 Biomechanical examination of the foot and lower extremity. In: Valmassey RL (ed) Clinical Biomechanics of the Lower Extremities. Mosby, St Louis, pp 131–148

Green DR, Carol A 1984 Plantar dominance. Journal of the American Podiatric Medical Association 74(2): 98–103

Gudas CJ 1979 Compression screw fixation in proximal first metatarsal osteotomies for metatarsus primus varus: initial observations. The Journal of Foot Surgery 18(1): 10–15

Hetherington VJ, Johnson RE, Albreitton JS 1990 Necessary dorsiflexion of the first metatarsophalangeal joint during gait. Journal of Foot Surgery 29(3): 218–222

Hice GA 1984 Orthotic treatment of feet having a high oblique midtarsal joint axis. Journal of the American Podiatric Medical Association 74(11): 577–582

Inman V 1976 Obliquity of the ankle axis in relation to the long axis of the tibia. The Joints of the Ankle. Williams & Wilkins, Baltimore, pp 26–28

Jack FA 1953 Naviculo-cuneiform fusion in the treatment of flat foot. Journal of Bone and Joint Surgery 35B(1): 75–82

Lang LMG 1987 The anatomy of the foot. Bailliere's Clinical Rheumatology 1(2): 215–240

Lang LMG 1990 A longitudinal study of growth and development in the lower limb. PhD Thesis, CNAA

Lindsjo U, Danckwardt-Lilliestrom, Sahlstedt B 1985 Measurement of the motor range in the loaded ankle. Clinical Orthopaedics and Related Research 199 October: 68–71

Lundberg A, Svensson OK, Bylund C, Goldie I, Selvik G 1989 Kinematics of the ankle/foot complex—Part 2: Pronation and supination. Foot & Ankle 9(5): 248–253

Manter JT 1941 Movements of the subtalar and transverse tarsal joints. Anatomy Record 80: 397–409

Minkowsky I, Minkowsky R 1996 The Spine: An integral part of the lower extremity. In: Valmassey RL (Ed) Clinical Biomechanics of the Lower Extremities. Mosby, St Louis, pp 95–112

Muller MJ, Host JV, Norton BJ 1993 Navicular drop as a composite measure of excessive pronation. Journal of the Podiatric Medical Association 83(4): 198–202

Perry J 1992 Ankle Foot Complex. Gait Analysis. Slack Incorporated Thorofare, pp. 51–87

Philips RD, Law EA, Ward ED 1996 Functional motion of the medial column joints of the foot during propulsion. Journal of the Podiatric Medical Association 86(10): 474–486

Phillips RD, Phillips RL 1983 Quantitative analysis of the locking position of the midtarsal joint. Journal of the American Podiatry Association 73(10): 518–522

Rogers MM, Cavanagh PR 1986 Glossary of biomechanical terms, concepts, and units. Physical Therapy 64(12): 1886–1902

Root ML, Orien WP, Weed JH 1971 Clinical Biomechanics — Volume I. Clinical Biomechanics Corporation, Los Angeles

Root ML, Orien WP, Weed JH 1977 Clinical Biomechanics — Volume II. Clinical Biomechanics Corporation, Los Angeles

Root ML, Weed JH, Sgarlato TE, Bluth DR 1966 Axis of motion of the subtalar joint. Journal of the American Podiatry Association 56(4): 149–156

Rose GK, Welton FA, Marshal T 1985 The diagnosis of flat foot in the child. Journal of Bone and Joint Surgery 67B(1): 71–78

Roukis TS, Scherer PR, Anderson CF 1996 Position of the first ray and motion of the first metatarsophalangeal joint. Journal of the American Podiatric Medical Association 86(11): 538–545

Southerland CC, Orien WP 1995 Seven theorems of compensation in the distal human lower extremity. The Lower Extremity 2(3): 173–186

Tachdjan MO 1985 The Child's Foot. Saunders, Philadelphia, pp 561–567

Valmassey RL 1996 Biomechanical evaluation of the child. In: Valmassey RL (ed) Clinical Biomechanics of the Lower Extremities. Mosby, St Louis, p. 243

Weed JH, Root M 1982 Direction and range of motion of the first ray. Journal of the American Podiatric Medical Association 72 (12): 600–605

Wernick J, Volpe RG 1996 Lower extremity function. In: Valmassey RL (Ed) Clinical Biomechanics of the Lower Extremities. Mosby, St Louis, pp 1–58

West SG 1987 A review of methods of obtaining foot loading data during walking. Chiropodist (3): 84–94

Wright DG, De sai ME, Henderson WH 1964 Action of the subtalar and ankle-joint complex during the stance phase of walking. Journal of Bone and Joint Surgery 46A(2): 361–383

7

Chiropractic manipulation of the foot: Diversified chiropractic techniques

D. J. Lawrence

Lincoln College of Postprofessional, Graduate and Continuing Education; Department of Editorial Review and Publication, National University of Health Sciences, Lombard, Illinois, USA.

There has been increasing acceptance and development of manual methods in providing for the needs of patients with musculoskeletal dysfunction. Several professions have helped fuel this growth, including the chiropractic profession. To date, there has been only a small amount of collaboration between chiropractors and physical therapists. This article provides a base foundation for one small part of general chiropractic practice, i.e. procedures used for manipulating the foot. Information is provided about the specific diagnostic procedures used by the chiropractic profession in assessing the joints and soft tissues of the foot, followed by descriptions of a number of chiropractic manipulative techniques drawn from the form of chiropractic in widest usage — diversified technique.

For each technique, information is provided on indications for use, patient position, therapist position, hand placements and procedure. In addition, a short discussion on the genesis of diversified technique is provided. *Manual Therapy* (2001) **6(2)**, 66–71

INTRODUCTION

As chiropractors gain greater acceptance, they continue to maintain and enhance their clinical diagnostic and assessment skills. Chiropractors utilize the same assessment procedures as other therapists, including standard case history, physical examination, laboratory examination, radiographic examination and various more specialized examinations (such as orthopaedic examination and neurological examination). They also utilize numerous procedures more unique to chiropractic. Taken as a whole, the information gathered from clinical examination will not only help to provide an appropriate and accurate diagnosis, but will lead the chiropractic to select the proper manipulative procedures needed to treat the patient. This article will examine some of those specialized diagnostic procedures and then use them to discuss one manipulative approach to managing the lower extremity.

Chiropractic examination, while certainly considering all aspects of the patient, focuses on assessing the spinal column, the peripheral joints, (where appropriate), and the nervous system. The goal is to identify any dysfunction, particularly of the joints. This may be referred to as subluxation, the vertebral subluxation complex or the vertebral subluxation syndrome (Bergmann & Finer 2000) From this dysfunction, the chiropractor can then assess the pathophysiological sequelae that arise from that dysfunction. In order to know which therapeutic procedures to use, it is necessary to identify the presence of joint dysfunction. A method of investigation has been developed by Bergmann et al (1993) that has helped to standardize the evaluation of joint structure and function. This system is used to determine what and how to perform a chiropractic manipulation.

This article will briefly examine the PARTS system (for definition see below) and then provide an overview of a specific system of chiropractic technique as it relates to manipulation in the lower extremity. The goal is to examine the types of technique in common use by chiropractors, and to that extent this is an overview or compendium of specific chiropractic procedures.

THE PARTS SYSTEM AND JOINT ASSESSMENT

Bergmann and Finer (2000) proposed the PARTS system as a multi-dimensional evaluative system that uses a number of different methods to gather information concerning joint function. PARTS consists of: Pain/tenderness; Asymmetry/alignment; Range of motion abnormality; Tone/texture/temperature of soft tissues; and Special tests. Given that examination of the musculoskeletal system cannot be accomplished by reliance upon a single method, the use of a multiple approach system is essential.

PAIN

Methods for identifying the presence of pain include observation, percussion, palpation and provocation. The pain itself is evaluated by its location, intensity and quality. Nearly all musculoskeletal conditions are accompanied by pain, and its evaluation is of critical importance in determining the diagnosis. The location of pain may be assessed through patient reporting, through pain drawings and through osseous and soft tissue palpation. Various tests can be used to reproduce pain, including most orthopaedic tests. While pain itself is a subjective finding, eliciting pain over osseous structures has been found to be a reliable indicator (Keating et al 1990). The presence of pain can also be seen as an indication of underlying joint dysfunction.

ASYMMETRY

Asymmetry must be noted on a number of levels, including global, regional or segmental. Asymmetry is assessed via postural examination, gait assessment, simple observation (i.e. on a radiograph or on a plumbline examination) and by static and motion palpation. Static palpation involves palpation of bony landmarks, and identification of joint malposition and tenderness/pain.

Postural spinal radiographic analysis, or spinography, is a set of procedures which require the analysis of radiographs taken while the patient is usually in the upright position; in this case the image demonstrates the effect of gravity on the spine. Of late, Harrison and colleagues (1999a, b) have invested a great deal of time and resources in studying posture radiographically, developing a model of the ideal normal spinal configuration, using engineering principles to do so.

RANGE OF MOTION ABNORMALITY

Motion palpation allows for identification of joint fixation, joint hypomobility or joint hyper-mobility, in active, passive and accessory joint motion. Typically, a loss of motion is noted at one level, and there is often compensatory increased motion at a level above or below that primary fixation. The main process involves examining the joint play in each joint, which is a necessary component of normal joint movement. The procedures were largely developed through the work of the Belgian chiropractors Gillet (1960) and Faye (1981). There are many methods of motion palpation, and these procedures are used not only in chiropractic but also in physiotherapy and osteopathy, among other disciplines.

Palpation for motion is the basis for most clinical decisions regarding when, where and how to manipulate a joint.

TISSUE TONE

The therapist must note any changes in soft tissues around the involved area. This may be done through observation, palpation, instrumentation and through tests of length and strength.

Bergmann and Finer (2000) note that:

Muscle tone is the result of continuous mild contraction of muscle dependent upon the integrity of nerves and their central connections with the complex properties of muscles such as contractibility, elasticity and extensibility. Normal muscles at rest possess resilience; thus, when joint movement passively stretches a muscle, a certain amount of involuntary resistance is encountered.

Obviously, normal muscle tone may be increased or decreased as a result of neurological input to the muscle. This may be a result of reflex changes or from a disease, injury or conditions affecting the region. Joint fixation may create abnormal neural reflex traffic, which may then cause hyper-tonicity or hypotonicity. This can be assessed through muscle-strength testing or dynamometry. Hypertonicity causes muscle spasticity, spasm and rigidity, while hypotonicity causes decreased resistance to passive movement and decreased strength. Muscles that are hypertonic may also exhibit hot spots on special tests such as thermograms, while the reverse is true in the case of hypotonicity. Electromyography (EMG) can provide more definitive data regarding muscle function; however, the value of surface EMG still remains questionable.

SPECIAL TESTS

Special tests refer to those procedures such as the supine leg length assessments needed for the Activator Technique (Fuhr et al 1996) or the arm fossa test arising from the sacro-occipital technique. Some of these tests have been investigated while others have not.

The above PARTS system can be applied to the spine or to the extremities equally well.

EXTREMITY TECHNIQUES

Diversified chiropractic technique was developed from the original work of Janse et al (1947). It is a measure of Janse's importance that the diversified technique remains the most widespread technique within the profession. In fact, the actual roots of the diversifed technique are rather difficult to locate, and certainly the work of pioneering medical manipulators may play a role, especially Mennell (1992) and Cyriax (1969). Most of the joint motion assessment procedures used today owe their origin to the work of Mennell. In addition, there is material that is believed to arise from the osteopathic profession; the term 'diversified' comes from the idea that the sources for these procedures are diverse in nature. Unlike other chiropractic techniques, diversified technique may be used within any chiropractic or manipulative system; it does not require its own parochial diagnostic methodologies. In this article, the procedures being discussed are derived from what is generally considered to be the standard compendium of diversified technique (Kirk et al 1985).

Methods for assessing specific joint motions have been well-established and can be found in virtually any text devoted to joint manipulation (Grieve 1984; DiGiovanna & Schiowitz 1997;

Berlinson 1989; Schafer & Faye 1989; Magee 1992; Mennell 1992; Plaugher 1993; Byfield 1996; Hammer 1999; Lewit 1999; Broome 2000). The general reasons for selecting any of the following procedures are found under the heading 'indications' in each technique description. In essence, the techniques are selected based upon clinical impressions, and are only part of a general therapeutic approach used by therapists. If used for specific conditions (i.e. pes planus, hallux rigidus or other conditions), these techniques are accompanied by the appropriate forms of physical modalities. This can vary widely depending upon the specific clinical situation, but may include such modalities as exercise, various forms of rehabilitation, electrical modalities (i.e. high-voltage pulsed galvanic current, interferential current, ultrasound etc.) Re-assessment is undertaken through clinical measures, via appropriate outcomes testing (i.e. visual analogue scale) and clinical results.

FOOT TECHNIQUES: PREMANIPULATIVE PROCEDURES

General foot technique

The general foot technique is used as a premanipulative procedure to loosen the soft tissues in the foot prior to performing an articular adjustment. In addition, it is used if there is foot strain, and is useful as an initial technique for patients unaccustomed to high-velocity, low-amplitude chiropractic adjustments. The patient lies supine and the therapist stands at the foot of the table. The therapist's hands are placed on either side of the midfoot, and are then alternately moved back and forth, thus everting and inverting the foot gently but quickly. This starts at a low rate and builds to a moderate rate. This procedure is typically performed for about 1 minute.

Metatarsal shear technique

This procedure is used to stretch adhesions formed between the metatarsal heads or to facilitate gentle motion when the metatarsal heads are not properly mobile. With the patient supine, the therapist places his or her thumbs on the sole of the foot, over the metatarsal head, and then wraps the fingers of both hands onto the dorsum of the foot. The motion is delivered by drawing one hand caudal while the other moves cephalad, in an alternating movement. This 'scissors' the metatarsal heads back and forth. The technique is modified when used for the great and second toe. In this case, the thenar pads of both hands are placed on the dorsum of the foot, wrapping the fingers around the sole of the foot. The same scissoring motion is then introduced. The modification takes into account the strength of the first toe and thus generalizes the movement to a greater extent. This is usually continued for 1–2 minutes.

Foot figure eight technique (Fig. 7.1)

This is generally felt to be a strong premanipulative procedure that loosens tissue, stretches adhesions, and also improves the circulation while reducing congestion and minor oedema. The therapist stands at the foot of the table while the patient lies supine. The therapist's contralateral hand cups the lateral ankle and calcaneum, holding it firmly from underneath to prevent the heel and ankle from moving during the procedure. The ipsilateral hand grasps the medial border of the foot, with the thumbs on the sole of the foot and the fingers wrapped around the dorsum.

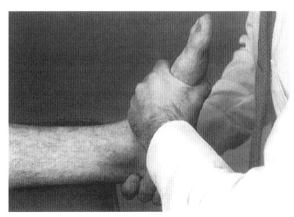

Figure 7.1 Foot figure eight. (Reprinted with permission of the National University of Health Sciences.)

The forefoot is then moved through a figure eight motion that has a medial to lateral orientation; the movement combines inversion with abduction followed by eversion with adduction. The technique is continued for 1–2 minutes.

Plantar compression technique

This procedure helps to stretch and mobilize the tissues located on the plantar surface of the foot, and can help to reduce swelling and oedema. It involves lifting the supine patient's foot and holding the foot with the cephalad hand while using the caudad hand to apply a stroking pressure on the sole of the foot for 1–2 minutes. This technique should not be used when plantar spurs are present, as compression of the foot will impinge upon the area where a spur exists.

Achilles tendon technique

This is a useful procedure to help stretch the Achilles tendon, to stretch adhesions that may have formed between the Achilles tendon and underlying structures, and to help reduce spasm in the gastrocnemius–soleus muscles. Again, the patient lies supine while the therapist stands at the side of the table. The straight leg is lifted with the caudal hand, which holds the medial calcaneum and is wrapped around the sole of the foot avoiding the patient's toes. The cephalad hand is placed so that it can monitor pressure in the medial insertion region of the gastrocnemius muscle. This prevents the muscle from being overstretched if it is tight, as may be the case in an elite athlete. The method of delivery involves careful application of pressure to dorsiflex the ankle, holding for a few seconds and then relaxing before repeating. This should not be performed rapidly but rather slowly and cautiously and repeated carefully over a 2–3 minute period.

Hallux mobilization technique

This technique is used to mobilize the great toe. It can be used either for mobilization or manipulation. In the former case, the therapist holds the medial margin of the foot just proximal to the first metatarsophalangeal joint. The other hands encircles the great toe and then moves it carefully through both spiral and figure eight motions for 1–2 minutes. In the case of manipulation, thrusts delivered in a medial direction can alternate with the mobilization.

FOOT TECHNIQUES: MANIPULATIVE PROCEDURES

Mortise separation technique (Fig. 7.2)

This procedure is used to mobilize the talocrural joint, and may also be used to help with biomechanical abnormalities arising from a subacute inversion ankle sprain. The patient lies supine with the practitioner kneeling at the foot of the table. Both hands grasp the foot, with the thumbs lying across the plantar surface of the foot and the fingers wrapped around the dorsum of the foot. To deliver the thrust, several manoeuvres must first be accomplished: the foot must be dorsiflexed (so that the ankle mortise is locked); the leg is then internally rotated (so that the hip is locked for the thrust that will follow); and then finally the foot is everted (which helps approximate the lateral collateral ligament of the ankle, and thus reduces the tension from the ligament). At this point, the thrust is delivered by pulling

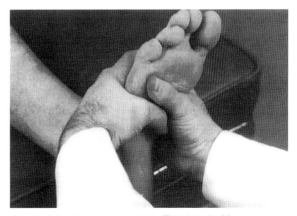

Figure 7.2 Mortise separation. (Reprinted with permission of the National University of Health Sciences.)

directly caudad towards the therapist. The procedure helps to re-establish proper alignment of the ankle mortise and its components.

Supine plantar cuneiform technique

This procedure is used for adjusting fixations of the cuneiforms and the navicular as well as for premanipulative mobilization. With the patient supine and the practitioner kneeling at the foot of the table, the hands grasp the foot so that the thumbs of each hand are placed on the involved area on the sole of the foot. The thumbs should point to the sides of the foot. The ankle is dorsiflexed and then everted; the thrust is delivered towards the practitioner and then the foot is inverted and another thrust is delivered.

Tarsal–metatarsal shear technique (Fig. 7.3)

This procedure will mobilize the cuneometatarsal and cubometatarsal joints. The patient lies supine with the knee flexed and only the heel on the table. The therapist stands at the side of the table. The therapist's cephalad hand grasps the foot firmly with the fingers pointing medially over the dorsum of the foot and the thumb pointing back towards the practitioner. The contact point is just proximal to the tarsal–metatarsal joints. In addition, the last two fingers wrap around the heel while the rest of the hand holds the foot in dorsiflexion. The therapist's caudal hand grasps the foot distal to the tarsal–metatarsal joint with the fingers pointing medially and thumb wrapped laterally. The hands then alternately shear the joint dorsal to plantar. The heel should be held against the table to provide stability.

Metatarsophalangeal flexion technique

There are numerous ways to mobilize the metatarsophalangeal (MP) joints in the foot. In this procedure, the index finger is hooked and held rigid just proximal to the MP joint on the plantar surface of the foot, while the thumb wraps

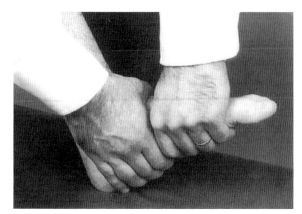

Figure 7.3 Tarsal–metatarsal shear. (Reprinted with permission of the National University of Health Sciences.)

over the toe to hold the dorsal proximal phalanx. The thrust is delivered by first flexing the toe to resistance and then quickly thrusting into further flexion. This can also be accomplished by using both hands as contacts on the patient's foot. The technique is further modified for the first MP joint. Here, the procedure requires the practitioner's thumbs to be interlaced over the dorsum of the great toe, one from inside the toe web and one from outside. Thus, the thumbs form an 'X' over the dorsum of the great toe while the rest of each hand is cupped underneath the great toe. After flexing the toe to resistance, the thrust is given into further flexion. This requires great care and caution, and should not be done if there are bunions present at the joint. The procedure may cause pain as a union located at the medial margin of the great toe will limit the amount of motion present.

Mortise shear technique (Fig. 7.4)

This procedure will mobilize the talocrural joint. The patient lies supine while the therapist stands at the side of the table. The cephalad hands grasps the ankle just above the ankle mortise, while the caudal hand holds it from below. The hands then alternately push and pull the contact points, creating shear movement at the ankle joint for 1–2 minutes. This can also be accomplished with the practitioner's hands reversed in position.

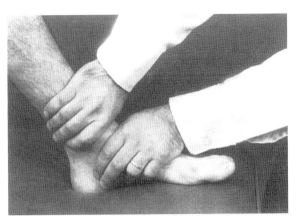

Figure 7.4 Mortise shear. (Reprinted with permission of the National University of Health Sciences.)

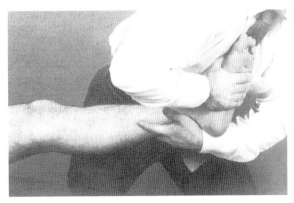

Figure 7.5 Medially subluxated talus technique. (Reprinted with permission of the National University of Health Sciences.)

Medially subluxated talus technique (Fig. 7.5)

This procedure is used to reduce medial subluxations or fixations of the talus. With the patient supine, and the therapist standing at the side of the table, the foot is held in the caudal hand so that the posterior distal calf is placed between the index and third finger and the heel is cradled on the distal forearm. The cephalad hand makes the contact, which involves placing the pisiform on the medial talar head, with the fingers over the medial border of the foot. The forearm is then moved medially so that the thrust, when it is delivered, is directed back towards the therapist.

Pisiform cuneiform technique

This procedure may be used to mobilize the cuneiforms and the navicular on the plantar surface of the foot. The patient lies prone, and the therapist stands at the side of the table. The therapist's caudal hand cradles the distal calf so that the ankle is held between the index and third finger. The contact is made by the cephalad hand. A pisiform contact is taken over the involved bone on the plantar surface of the foot. The fingers hold the medial border of the foot to provide stability. The elbow of the contact arm is held rigid, and the thrust is delivered with a quick thrust toward the floor, with a slight scooping motion.

Pes planus technique

This procedure is used to elevate the medial longitudinal arch. The patient lies supine while the practitioner stands at the side of the table. The cephalad hand has its thumb and index finger over the calcaneum near the insertion of the Achilles tendon. The caudal hand grasps the lateral border of the foot so that the fingers point away from the practitioner on the dorsal surface of the foot. The thrust is delivered by using the cephalad hand to lift the calcaneus while the caudal hand everts the forefoot. This is delivered in a smooth fashion rather than with a forceful articular thrust.

Plantar snap technique (Fig. 7.6)

This procedure is used for plantar fixations or subluxations of any tarsal bone. With the patient prone, the therapist stands at the foot of the table and crosses the thumbs of each hand over the involved tarsal bone so that they form an 'X'. The hands grasp the foot firmly. The ankle is then plantar flexed and a quick downward thrust is delivered to the involved bone.

General calcaneal technique

This technique will mobilize the calcaneum. The patient is again prone with the knee flexed and held so that the patient's foot is placed against the

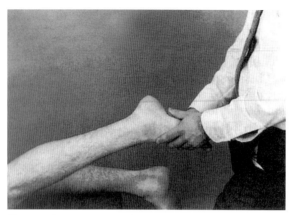

Figure 7.6 Plantar snap. (Reprinted with permission of the National University of Health Sciences.)

therapist's abdomen. Both hands are then placed in such a manner as to cup the patient's heel, and the manoeuvre requires the heel to be moved gently through a figure eight motion.

CONCLUSION

The intent of this article is to provide a firm foundation in chiropractic manipulative and pre-manipulative techniques for the foot as well as an understanding of the diagnostic systems unique to the chiropractic profession. To that end a compendium of techniques and procedures have been described, drawn from the tradition of diversified chiropractic technique. As the various professions that provide manipulative care begin to collaborate more in various settings, the time has come for sharing ideas and practices; i.e. to put the patient ahead of professional self-interest and parochial economic interests. Only by studying what we each offer can we best serve the patients who seek our service.

REFERENCES

Bergmann T, Finer BA 2000 Joints assessment—PARTS. Topics in Clinical Chiropractcs 7: 1–10

Bergmann T, Peterson D, Lawrence D 1993 Chiropractic Technique. Churchill Livingstone, New York

Berlinson G 1989 Precis de Medecine Osteopathetique rachidienne. Editions Maloine, Paris

Broome RT 2000 (ed) Chiropractic Peripheral Joint technique. Butterworth-Heinemann, Oxford

Byfield D 1996 Chiropractic Manipulative Skills. Butterworth-Heinemann, Oxford

Cyriax J 1969 Textbook of Orthopedic Medicine. Williams and Wilkins, Baltimore, MD

DiGiovanna EL, Schiowitz S 1997 An Osteopathic Approach to Diagnosis and Treatment. Lippincott-Raven, Philadelphia, PA

Faye LJ 1981 Motion palpation of the spine: from MPI notes and review of the literature. Motion Palpation Institute, Huntington Beach, CA

Fuhr AW, Colloca CJ, Green JR, Keller TS 1996 Activator methods — Chiropractic Technique. Mosby Year Book, St. Louis, MO

Gillet H 1960 Vertebral fixations: an introduction to movement palpation. Annals of the Swiss Chiropractic Association 1:30

Grieve GP 1984 Mobilisation of the Spine, 4th edn. Churchill Livingstone, New York

Hammer WI 1999 Functional Soft Tissue Examination and Treatment by Manual Methods: New Perspectives, 2nd edn. Aspen Publishing, Gaithersburg, MD

Harrison DE, Cailliet R, Harrison DD, Troyanovich SJ, Harrison SO 1999a A review of biomechanics of the central nervous system, part I: spinal canal deformations due to changes in posture. Journal of Manipulative Physiological Therapeutics 22: 227–234

Harrison DE, Cailliet R, Harrison DD, Troyanovich SJ, Harrison SO 1999b A review of biomechanics of the central nervous system. Part II: strains in the spinal cord from postural loads. Journal of Manipulative Physiological Therapeutics 22: 322–332

Janse JJ, Houser RH, Wells RF 1947 Chiropractic principles and Technic. National College of Chiropractic, Chicago, IL

Keating JC, Bergmann T, Jacobs GE, Finer BA, Larson K 1990 Interexaminer reliability of eight evaluative dimensions of lumbar segmental abnormality. Journal of Manipulative Physiological Therapeutics 13: 463–470

Kirk CR, Valvo NL, Lawrence DJ 1985 States Manual of Spinal, Pelvic and Extravertebral Technic. National College of Chiropractic, Lombard, IL

Lewit K 1999 Manipulative Therapy in Rehabilitation of the Locomotor System, 3rd edn. Butterworth–Heinemann, Oxford

Magee DJ 1992 Orthopedic Physical Assessment, 2nd edn. WB Saunders, Philadelphia, PA

Mennell JM 1992 The Musculoskeletal System: Differential Diagnosis from Symptoms and Physical signs. Aspen Publishing, Gaithersburg, MD

Plaugher G 1993 (Ed) Textbook of Clinical Chiropractic: a Specific Biomechanical Approach. Williams and Wilkins, Baltimore, MD

Schafer RC, Faye LJ 1989 Motion Palpation and Chiropractic Technic: Principles of Dynamic Chiropractic. Motion Palpation Press, Huntington Beach, CA

General

SECTION CONTENTS

8

Gait analysis in the therapeutic environment

F.J. Coutts
Department of Health Sciences, University of East
London, Stratford, UK

Gait analysis is one aspect of the overall assessment of any patient with a movement disorder. Loss of walking ability is often a major issue for the patient, thus justifying the length of time that should be spent in establishing gait problems and planning re-education. Biomechanical measures of kinematics, kinetics and electromyographical activity are essential to give a complete picture of the specific gait characteristics (Perry 1992; Whittle 1996b). However, observational analysis remains the most commonly used tool in the therapeutic situation (Patla et al 1987). Reliability of observational analysis is poor (Krebs et al 1985) and therapists should be encouraged to use objective measures to give a more representative account of the gait pattern. A systematic approach to data collection and recording should be adopted and the key kinematic data of walking, including velocity, stride length, base of support and joint angles, should be collected in order to provide a baseline on which to measure clinical effectiveness. Valid outcome measures must be established to evaluate gait effectively to afford therapists the ability to assess their treatment of gait deviations. An understanding of biomechanical terminology is essential to aid the selection of appropriate gait analysis tools and for interpretation of the results. *Manual Therapy* (1999) **4(1)**, 2–10

INTRODUCTION

Gait assessment and analysis is an inherent component in the evaluation of patients with movement disorders. The extent and complexity of the measurement depends on the experience of and resources available to the therapist, but subjective observation is the most common approach used in the clinical setting. The literature suggests that the term 'clinical gait analysis' is associated with the work of gait laboratories and does not reflect the assessment undertaken in the therapy clinics or in the patient's home (Whittle 1996a; Davis 1997). It is with this in mind that this article presents the key elements and history of gait analysis and explores the types of assessment that can be used in the therapeutic environment.

Rose (1983) suggests that 'gait assessment' is a problem-solving exercise that involves the complete process of subjective and objective evaluation of gait, physical examination of the patient and a review of the treatment decisions undertaken in the clinical situation. Whittle (1996a), however, describes 'gait analysis' as the evaluation of human motion in gait laboratories and may be regarded as a special test. The difference is historical and there is no doubt that prior to the evolution of computerized motion analysis systems the only form of 'gait analysis' was observation and simple temporal spatial measures in the therapeutic situation.

Gait analysis in the laboratory consists of the collection of biomechanical data [Kinemetic, Kinetic and Electromyography (EMG)] and is often accompanied by videotaping to give an overall interpretation of the quality of the patients' movement capability. Kinematics is the study of movement, requiring the recording of time and distance data, joint angles and accelerations over time (temporal–spatial data). Kinetics is predominantly concerned with the forces and moments existing between the foot and the ground and can also interpret the position of the ground reaction force vector relative to each joint (Whittle 1996b). EMG records the electrical muscle activity during movement and can be measured via fine wire, needle or surface electrodes (Perry 1992; Whittle 1996b).

Gait assessment measures effects not causes (Rose 1983) and there has to be an understanding of the whole perspective and interpretation with clinical problem solving before the patient can be assisted. Therefore, gait assessment is one part of the overall patient evaluation and further tests may be required to establish the treatment protocol, e.g laboratory gait analysis, X-ray or magnetic resonance imaging scans.

HISTORY

The first reported studies of human walking were undertaken in the 1940s and 1950s in California (Inman et al 1981) using cine film to capture the moving figure. Following the development of computerized systems with infra-red or video-based cameras (e.g. the Vicon System, Oxford Metrics Limited, Oxford, UK), the process of recording and analysis was made much quicker and easier in the late 1970s and early 1980s.

There are many visible or infra-red three-dimensional motion analysis systems available from the commercial market (Vicon System, Oxford Metrics Limited, Oxford, UK; Elite Bioengineering Technology Systems, Milan, Italy; Kinemetrix, MIE Limited, Leeds, UK; Coda, Charnwood Dynamics Limited, UK), but costs are high for the purchase, upkeep and running of any of the systems.

Also at this time three-dimensional force plates were being developed and together with the use of EMG, which evolved in the 1940s and 1950s, fully integrated gait analysis could be undertaken (Whittle 1996a). Thus, from the 1970s onwards laboratory gait analysis has been used as an evaluation and research tool, but still remains limited to a small number of specialist centres.

Several centres are renowned for their novel work in gait analysis, but Jaquelin Perry (Downey, CA), David Sutherland (San Diego CA), Jim Gage (Newington), David Winter (Canada) and Gordon Rose (Oswestry, UK) were the main contributors. As a result of their contributions many more gait analysis laboratories were established in numerous countries and the biomechanical understanding of gait, both normal and pathological, became more widespread.

Interpretation of biomechanical data is complex, time consuming and not readily understood by most therapists, and this has added to the difficulties of transferring the knowledge gained from the laboratory to the therapy situation. Laboratory analysis, however, with all its limitations, remains the 'gold' standard and a good understanding of the biomechanics of normal gait is essential if proficient therapeutic gait analysis is to be undertaken. Several papers are available to assist this understanding (Rose 1983; Mendeiros 1984; Yack 1984; Bowker & Messenger 1988; Whittle 1996a; Kopf et al 1998).

There is no doubt that gait analysis in the laboratory provides an abundance of excellent information about the performance of the activity, but unfortunately it is costly, inconvenient and highly sophisticated and is, therefore, not readily available to most clinicians (Krebs et al 1985). The use of gait laboratories has, therefore, been limited to the analysis of more complex problems, e.g. diagnosis and treatment evaluation of children and adolescents with cerebral palsy, prosthetic development and adult neurological pathologies (Davis 1997).

Shores (1980), Little (1981), Robinson & Smidt (1981), and Clarkson (1983) all report simple measures to be used in the therapeutic context, which require no more than space, a stopwatch and recording materials. The advent of video (Kinsman 1986; Stuberg et al 1988; Wall 1991) and computers (Wall & Crosbie 1996, 1997) has helped to transfer the use of easy, but more sophisticated data collection, to the therapeutic environment to capture real-time gait events. Unfortunately, the use of either video or computers is still not common practice in the therapeutic environment in the UK.

NORMAL GAIT

The biomechanics of 'normal' gait are presented in many texts from a brief overview, e.g. Craik and Oatis (1985), to the excellent book by Whittle (1996b), thorough but less complex.

This article will not discuss normal gait data and uses the definitions of the phases of gait that are taken from Rancho Los Amigos Medical Center (1989) and Perry (1992). The main phases of the cycle and their definitions are to be found in Table 8.1.

Table 8.1 Phases of the gait cycle. (Los Amigos Research and Education Institute, Rancho Los Amigos Medical Center, Downey, CA [1989] Observational Gait Analysis Handbook.)

	Phase of the gait cycle	Defintion
Stance	Initial contact	The moment when the foot hits the ground
Stance	Loading response	The body weight is transferred onto the lead limb
Stance	Midstance	The body progresses over a single stable limb
Stance	Terminal stance	Progression over the stance limb continues and the body moves ahead of the limb and weight is transferred onto the forefoot
Transition	Pre-swing	A rapid unloading occurs as weight is transferred to the other limb
Swing	Initial swing	The thigh advances as the foot is lifted clear of the floor
Swing	Mid-swing	The thigh continues to advance and the knee having reached maximum flexion now extends, keeping the foot clear of the floor
Swing	Terminal swing	The knee extends and the limb prepares to take the load at initial contact

GAIT ANALYSIS IN THE THERAPEUTIC ENVIRONMENT

When deciding the type of the gait assessment to be used the therapist must ask the specific question – Why am I doing this gait assessment? There are many answers to the question including:

1. To give an overall impression of the performance
2. To allow the patient to become aware of specific gait problems
3. To assess the position of the foot in the stance phase
4. To measure the speed and distance of walking
5. To measure overall fitness.

In each therapeutic situation the answer will differ and the therapist needs to have a range of skills and tools to measure the effectiveness of treatment.

Observational skills and videoing may be the only tools required to answer the first of these two questions, but how adequate would they be for specific impairment issues of gait?

Observation and subjective recording of gait will never be totally superseded as the mainstay of gait assessment in the therapeutic environment because of ease of use, but the therapist should be aware of all the limitations and the alternatives available to them.

OBSERVATIONAL ANALYSIS

Global terms to identify characteristics, e.g. 'antalgic gait', have been used as a quick summary of the most easily observed gait deformities, but they can only give a quick overall impression and lack depth of analysis (Yack 1984). Observation and subjective recording of gait are the mainstay of gait assessment in the therapeutic environment (Yack 1984; Krebs et al 1985), although there is no knowledge of the level or extent of use in the UK.

Poor observational ability, personal bias, lack of experience, poor training of the technique and limitations of visual perception flaw observational analysis (Krebs et al 1985). Added to this there is no agreement on what to assess in observation analysis. Therefore, it is not surprising that poor intra- and inter-rater reliability has been found by many researchers (Goodkin & Diller 1973; Krebs et al 1985; Patla et al 1987; Eastlack et al 1991).

While researching observational skills using videotaping, Krebs et al (1985) found a total agreement of 67.5% when three therapists assessed the gait of 15 children. Likewise, Eastlack et al (1991) found only slight to moderate agreement (κ 0.11–0.52) when 54 therapists assessed three patients with rheumatoid arthritis. In patients following stroke, Hughes and Bell (1994) ascertained significant agreement between three raters for the swing phase parameters of gait but not for the stance phase or for the overall description of the gait characteristics.

There is limited literature on the level of observational gait assessment skills without the use of video, but there is no doubt that without video

playback facilities these skills would be far more unreliable.

Although observation of specific parameters may be flawed, observation can provide the therapist with a general impression of the quality of movement and help to assess the overall functional walking ability of the patient, for example: how the patients interact with their environment; how they manoeuvre around obstacles; how they use walking aids; whether they are easily distracted; whether they can handle different environments (outdoors, slopes, rough ground, busy streets, etc.).

This material is valuable and provides 'functional' information. Videotaping in these environments is difficult so the therapist must have specific objectives of observation and these will differ depending on the level of ability of the patient.

As the overall description and recording of abnormal gait is fundamentally flawed, a standardized framework, recording format and acceptance of terminology, are all required to enhance clinical judgement. One such system is that defined in the *Observational Gait Analysis Handbook* (Rancho Los Amigos Medical Centre, 1989), further examples will be given later.

Currently, observational analysis on its own is insufficiently reliable to be clinically acceptable. Either training and practice of observation must be enhanced or observation should be augmented by objective tests of gait to measure clinical effectiveness.

STRUCTURE OF GAIT ASSESSMENT IN THE THERAPEUTIC ENVIRONMENT

As the therapeutic situation is extremely variable there is no standard structure for gait assessment but several points have to be considered.

VIDEO TAPING

Video taping of the gait assessment will enhance the observational skills of the therapists by allowing repeated viewing at slower speeds or freezing specific frames for closer inspection. The advantage to the patient of videoing the event is that they should be less fatigued, as the number of repetitions will reduce, and that they will see a recording of their performance and become aware of any deviations. The disadvantage of any observation, but especially with the presence of video cameras, is that the patient can be acutely aware of the 'performance' and gait pattern modification can occur to put on a good show (Rose 1983). Securing privacy within the room, keeping cameras as unobtrusive as possible and ensuring that the patient is at ease will assist in obtaining 'normal' movement. Standardization of the position of the video camera(s) (usually 90° to the sagittal or frontal plane), the 'walkway', the level of light and the general environment will all help to allow comparison of findings from one day to the next and focus the eye of the reviewer. For the more detailed assessment of gait, more objective measures have to be taken.

OBJECTIVE ASSESSMENT

Objective measures fall into several categories:

1. Measurement of time and distance data
2. Measurement of joint and limb motion
3. Measurement of overall walking ability

TIME AND DISTANCE DATA

Walking tests are now an accepted part of the measurement of gait (Butland et al 1981; Singh et al 1992; Wade 1992). The walking test can either be set by time or distance, i.e. the 2-, 6- and 12-minute walking test or the 3- or 10-metre walking test. Walking tests have been used to assess general respiratory fitness (Singh 1992), pre- and postoperative performance in patients with orthopaedic problems (McNicol et al 1980, 1981) or overall gait disability in the neurological area. The 10-metre timed walk test has been used extensively in the assessment of neurological gait (Wade 1992). Smith (1993) suggests that in laboratory assessment of gait only one walking trial is necessary for intra-patient assessment but the mean of three trials should be used for inter-patient assessment.

The test requires that either the time taken to walk a set distance is recorded, or that the total distance walked over a set time is recorded to give an indication of the walking velocity and cadence. Many researchers and clinicians have used gait velocity to reflect change in gait performance as a result of treatment (e.g. Robinson & Smidt 1981; McNicol et al 1980, 1981; Wade 1992). There is a significant correlation between the walking velocity and many other components of gait, e.g. balance ability, quadriceps strength and length of the tendo achilles (Steadman et al 1997a) and, therefore, velocity is often used as a clinical outcome measure. Wade et al (1987) also demonstrated that walking velocity correlated with the clinical assessment of the gait pattern following stroke.

The number of steps or strides can also be counted to measure cadence and there are recognized normal values for these measures (Whittle 1996b).

The longer walking tests (either time or distance) should be used to assess the gait of the more able patients (Butland et al 1981; Gulmans et al 1996). The 3-minute test has been used in the elderly (Wolfson et al 1990) and was found to have low variability within one session and was repeatable over 24 hours in elderly patients (Worsfold & Simpson 1996). The greatest advantage of this test is that it can be used in both the clinical and the home environment, without adaptation.

ENVIRONMENT FOR THE WALKING TEST

Ideally the environment for the walking test should be well lit, quiet, and cleared of all equipment. The walking space should ideally be 10 metres in length (Robinson & Smidt 1981) and allow the therapist room to move to the front, back and side of the patient (Whittle 1996b). Any distractions to the patient should be removed, e.g. mirrors, people, and video cameras should be kept as far removed from the walking field as possible. Discrete distance markers on the floor or wall may help if a timed walk is to be undertaken and chairs should be provided at the ends of the walkway.

Robinson & Smidt (1981) recommend a more structured 10-metre walkway with adhesive tape applied to the floor to mark out a grid of 10 metres × 0.3 metres with numbered transverse strips at 3 cm intervals. Although this allows ease of collection of stride length and step length the 'grid' may guide the patient and influence performance. Worsfold and Simpson (1996) noted that patients who declared a fear of falling and difficulty walking both indoors and outdoors were more at ease walking in the corridor than in any other environment. Subconscious gait changes may occur in different environments and may be influenced by cueing, such as gridlines or narrow corridor.

Stride and step length can only be measured if there is a representation of foot contact and usually heel strike is taken. Recording onto a dictaphone whenever the patient's foot makes contact with a measured point on the floor grid can provide the number of steps/strides taken, step/stride length and the distance from the starting point. Other measures can also be used to measure step/stride length:

1. Simple methods of gait analysis
   • Footprint analysis (Shores 1980; Clarkson 1983; Kippen 1993, Volpon 1994)
   • Event markers, e.g. pens attached to the heels, talcum powder on floor, sand
   • Ticker tape analysis (Law & Minns 1989)
   • Calculation: overall length walked divided by the number of strides will give the mean overall stride length, or the number of steps will give the mean overall step length (McNicol et al 1980, 1981). This technique is not as accurate as the direct measurement of the step and stride length
2. Complex and more expensive methods
   • Instrumented shoes, foot switches (Yack 1984; Rowe et al 1989; Whittle 1996b)
   • Pressure mats or walkways systems (Silvino et al 1980; Wall et al 1981; SMS Health Care Ltd 1998)
   • Personal computer based systems (Wall 1991; Wall & Crosbie 1996, 1997)
   • Optoelectric Motion Analysis Systems (infra-red or visible light) (Whittle 1996a; Davis 1997)

The other distance parameter that can be measured is the dynamic width of support or walking base (normal 50–100 mm) (Whittle 1996b), i.e. the horizontal distance between the centre of the feet during double support time. The static base of support measured from the standing posture just prior to walking (87.5 mm [Perry 1992]), is only a true representation of base of support during the midstance phase of gait. As the width of the base of support increases, dynamic balance ability increases (Winter et al 1990). The wider the dynamic base of support the less the subject has to use muscle control at the hips and ankles and vice versa (Perry 1992). Alternatively the patient may not widen the base of support but may lower the centre of mass by flexing the knees on walking. The base of support will look normal but comparison of knee flexion during standing and walking will indicate the problem.

JOINT AND LIMB MOTION

Joint and limb motion can only be a subjective observational guess unless electrogoniometers (Rowe et al 1989) or an optoelectric motion analysis system is available in the therapeutic situation.

When observing limb segment motion, several parameters can be estimated:

• Range and timing of motion
• Starting position of the joint and limb segments (including deformities)
• Acceleration of the limb segments.

Measuring joint angles directly from the television screen (from freeze frame on videotape) is prone to error and, therefore, cannot give true objective data. The advent of the video-based computer system via the ordinary personal computer means cheaper and easier objective measures are starting to be available in the therapeutic environment in the UK (Wall & Crosbie 1996, 1997).

The observation of joint motion or limb segment position is particularly difficult and unreliable without the use of videotape. A video recorder with a freeze frame and jog per frame facility is also preferable, allowing the therapist time to study the position of the body or limb segments. A systematic approach to joint and limb motion is required for enhancing observational techniques and for consistency of results. Patla et al (1987) report that the 22 therapists they studied predominantly used a variety of starting points when studying specific body segments, e.g. foot to head, hip to foot. Once the therapists had established a systematic approach, they kept to it. There is no evidence in the literature to indicate whether the observer should start at the foot and work up to the head or vice versa, or concentrate on the lower limb before the trunk. Whichever approach is used a routine should be established, practised and used for all patients. Ideally all planes of motion should be observed, but realistically only the frontal and sagittal plane can be assessed. Krebs et al (1985) report that sagittal plane movements are more reliable than frontal or transverse, and that movements at the larger joints, i.e. hip and knee, are more reliable than movements at the foot and ankle.

The use of visual cues such as skin markers (removable pen marks or small 1 cm adhesive discs) on bony prominences will assist the observation of the joint movement. Specifically the acromion, anterior superior iliac spine, greater trochanter, lateral femoral condyle, lateral malleolus and fifth metatarsal head are the points of choice but additional markers can be placed on the posterior superior iliac spines, anterior thigh and anterior shank to assist observation of rotation (Perry 1992). Obviously this requires that the patient is suitably undressed and markers should contrast the skin colour.

Vertical lines, i.e. wall bars or a grid on the wall, may also help with recognizing joint position and the position of the trunk relative to the vertical (Kinsman 1986). The observation of standing posture from the frontal and sagittal planes will help assess the static posture and will indicate any change in spinal postures or deformities caused by dynamic loading, such as valgus/varus, hip abductor weakness (Trendelenberg test) and increased lumbar lordosis.

Patla et al (1987) reported that the majority of the therapists questioned looked only at the stance phase of gait for patients with back, ankle and knee problems, whilst both stance and swing were evaluated in those with hip problems. It can only be presumed that this was because the therapists did not think that gait deviations might occur in the swing phase of patients with back, ankle and knee problems.

This is unacceptable and all the limb segments should be observed in both the swing and stance phases of gait. For the therapist to recognize the specific difficulties at individual joints, knowledge of the phases of gait and the 'normal' values for starting positions and joint ranges during the gait cycle for specific age groups is essential (Sutherland et al 1980; Winter et al 1987; Whittle 1996b).

Table 8.2 outlines the mean range of movement in the sagittal plane that is required for normal walking.

Some of the angles in the table, e.g. hip extension in terminal stance, may appear large but any one angle will depend on the position of the long axis. In this case the trunk axis was taken as the true vertical plane and the leg axis as the line of the femur, giving a relative position of 20° of extension. In observational analysis it is common to take the trunk axis as the line from the greater trochanter to the acromion, therefore the hip angle could appear to be reduced at terminal stance. If the trunk is flexed, the hip will appear to be in a lesser degree of extension (Fig. 8.1), but the relative position to the vertical is still 20° extension.

Therefore, when observing gait the therapist must think about the measurement axes. Except for the hip joint, the axes will normally be the lines bisecting the length of the bone. Thus as the thigh and lower leg move there will be a relative change in angle at the knee joint. At initial contact the ankle joint is in the neutral position with the knee in neutral and the hip at 25° of flexion (Rancho Los Amigos Medical Center 1989), although on observation the ankle may appear dorsiflexed because of the relative knee position. Loading response differs from initial contact because the knee has flexed to 15° and the ankle is now in 10° plantar flexion (Rancho Los Amigos Medical Center 1989). The ankle looks as if it has not moved from the neutral position but is in plantar flexion because the tibia is still behind the axis of

Table 8.2 Range of motion summary in the sagittal plane measured in degrees. (Rancho Los Amigos Medical Center [1989] Observational Gait Analysis Handbook. Downey, CA. Los Amigos Research and Education Institute.)

Phase of the gait cycle	Stance Initial contact	Stance Loading response	Stance Midstance	Stance Terminal stance	Transition Pre-swing	Swing Initial swing	Swing Midswing	Swing Terminal swing
Pelvis	5 Forward rotation	5 Forward rotation	0	5 Backward rotation	5 Backward rotation	5 Backward rotation	0	5 Forward rotation
Hip Joint	25 Flexion	25 Flexion	0	20 Extension	0	15 Flexion	25 Flexion	25 Flexion
Knee Joint	0	15 Flexion	0	0	40 Flexion	60 Flexion	25 Flexion	0
Ankle Joint	0	10 PF	5 DF	10 DF	20 PF	10PF	0	0
Toes	0	0	0	30 MTP Extension	60 MTP Extension	0	0	0

PF = Plantar flexion; DF = Dorsiflexion; MTP = Metatarsophalangeal joint.

motion (ankle joint) whilst the foot is in contact with the ground.

The skill of assessing joint motion by observation is to know the normal ranges, to monitor the position of the limbs relative to the joints and to be able to describe the axes of the angles being monitored.

Therapists need assistance in recognizing the relative motion of the limb segments and thus video can help. By freezing the frame of the video at the point in the gait cycle being assessed the position of the limb segment can be viewed and compared against a vertical line dropped from the top of the television monitor. For example, when measuring hip movement in the sagittal plane, if a vertical line is placed near the hip joint centre (approximately the greater trochanter), then the relative position of the lower limb segments and trunk can be taken from this. This can also be done in the frontal plane view, but the vertical line is more difficult to place because there is no definitive point of rotation. This technique is purely to help judge the relative positions of the limb segments not to measure the actual joint angle.

Assessing the acceleration or timing of the limb segments is enhanced by video taping because the tape can be slowed down to observe more time-specific changes such as foot drop or knee instability at terminal swing/initial contact.

Changes in acceleration or timing of the limb segments are predominantly due to loss (reduction in strength and/or recruitment) or increase of muscle control (spasm, overactivity or spasticity). EMG can be used to help record which muscle is working and the level, timing and extent of muscle activity in the dynamic situation (Perry 1992).

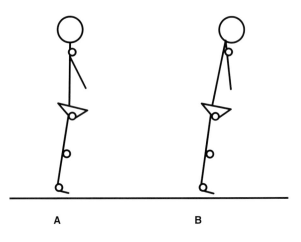

A B

Figure 8.1 Relative hip position to the vertical. (A) Vertical trunk, 20° apparent hip extension, 0° knee and 10° dorsiflexion of ankle. (B) Flexed trunk, 20° apparent hip extension, 0° knee, 10° dorsiflexion of ankle.

MEASURE OF OVERALL WALKING ABILITY

Mulder et al (1998) reviewed the literature available on gait assessment and noted that the majority of measures were used to assess impairment and simple motor functions rather than the 'disability' of walking. Disability scales should be based on how the patient perceives their ability to walk but are often completed by the therapist or carer who obviously report what they feel or observe about the overall disability. The Rivermead Mobility Index has been used as a measure of walking disability (Wade 1992; Steadman et al 1997a) but there remains a lack of information on gait disability in general, which requires further investigation.

Measures of respiratory function can be used as a global indicator of the effect an altered walking pattern has on energy expenditure and disability. These are often costly and laboratory-based but indices of overall cardiorespiratory function may be useful. The Physiological Cost Index (PCI) is one such index and can be calculated by the difference of the end of walk to resting heart rate divided by the speed.

$$\frac{PCI}{(beats/metre)} = \frac{\text{HR at end of walk} - \text{Resting HR}}{(beats/minute) \quad (beats/minute)}$$
$$\text{Speed (metres/minute)}$$

This gives a global indication of the energy expenditure of walking and does not require expensive equipment. The index is sensitive to change and has been used in both adults (Nene 1993) and children (Butler et al 1984) and validated as a comparative index of energy cost (McGregor 1981). However, this is not a true measure of the disability of walking; one such measure is the 'patient perception' questionnaire used to assess walking disability in patients following stroke (Steadman et al 1997b). This simple questionnaire correlated significantly with walking velocity, Berg balance scores and the results of the Rivermead Mobility Index, indicating that the perceptions of patients with moderate to severe walking disability gave an indication to their overall physical performance

(Steadman et al 1997b). Further investigations need to be done in this field to validate measures of walking disability.

RECORDING

If objective measures have been recorded, e.g. gait velocity, timing, distance and step length, then there is no need for a specific recording format to be used, so long as all the parameters are recorded clearly. However, when recording the impressions from observation the therapist can make a choice from a number of recording formats depending on how detailed the observation or measurement has been. Patla et al (1987) questioned 22 therapists on their gait analysis procedures, reporting that 'Unfortunately, after doing such a detailed examination, the final report takes the form of a single comment'. It is easy to make and record a quick and simple overall impression but this does not give a suitable outcome measure, only a subjective qualitative opinion. It may be easy to interpret this information at the time of writing, but at a later date the words could be meaningless and the overall interpretation may change. When describing the relevant components therapists tend to look at, and record, the easier global temporal–spatial parameters of 'width of base of support, torso positioning, symmetry and foot placement, stride length and cadence' (Patla et al 1987).

Examples of the charts available for recording these impressions include:

- Recording the estimated range of motion overall or at the appropriate phase of gait (Reimers 1972; Patla et al 1987)
- Ticking a box if the there is a loss or gain of motion, or for specific gait deviations (Rancho Los Amigos Medical Center 1989)
- Using an ordinal scale to record the quality and/or quantity of the gait deviation (e.g. Lower Limb Orthotics 1981; Krebs et al 1985; Eastlack et al 1991; Hughes & Bell, 1994; Lord et al 1998).

Which chart to use will depend on the question asked in the first instance. The simplest format is to record all the phases of the gait cycle and write down the main abnormal components observed. This only gives a global view and is open to misinterpretation if normal gait terminology and data are not up to date. The observational gait analysis (OGA) form (Rancho Los Amigos Medical Center 1989) requires the therapist to indicate if there is a gait deformity present at any of the joints, through any phase of the gait cycle. If there is a deformity present then this will indicate either a major or minor effect on walking ability; the chart has been colour-coded to help in this decision. The successful use of the Rancho Los Amigos OGA form requires both practice and a complete understanding of the terminology, as it is complex and time consuming. The team at Rancho Los Amigos has developed a complete observational package and the OGA form is only one part of this. The package helps the therapist to understand the implications of the gait deformities and the causes of these, thus aiding problem solving in gait analysis. This type of recording means that the therapist must have a full understanding of normal kinematic gait data and be conversant with the terminology used in the form.

The commonest means of recording gait deformity is use of the ordinal scale. The therapist is asked to indicate from a list of possibilities whether a gait deformity is present, and the extent of its presence. Krebs et al (1985) used the symbols 0 for normal gait, + for just noticeably abnormal gait and ++ for very noticeably abnormal gait. Eastlack et al (1991) used the scale 1 = inadequate, N = normal and E = excessive. The main problem with these scales is the lack of specific definitions, for example what does 'just noticeably abnormal' or 'inadequate' mean. Lord et al (1998) developed a form using a 4-point ordinal scale, giving very

clear definitions of each component of the form. The definitions are based on the normal position of the joint and by reference to them the therapist records the gait deviation as being 'normal, mild, moderate or severe'. Although not all points on the scale have been defined there is a standardized definition from which the therapist can make a judgement.

One recording format will not be acceptable in all therapeutic environments, but whatever the choice it must represent the answer to the question asked at the start – Why am I doing the gait assessment?

CONCLUSION

Assessment of gait is an important part of the vast array of investigations that the therapist has to undertake and it is often the test that is regarded as being easy to do and understand. Indeed, most therapists feel confident about their ability to assess gait (Patla et al 1987). This is not borne out by the literature and a systematic approach to both objective data collection and recording of subjective opinion is essential. Video analysis can assist the efficiency of the analysis both for the therapist and the patient.

As with all practice, if measurement of treatment change is performed in a systematic and objective system then good outcome measures will follow. Much more work is needed on the assessment of gait in the therapeutic situation for true outcome measures to be established and this must start with the recognition that our skills of gait assessment need to be enhanced and practised.

REFERENCES

Bowker P, Messenger N 1988 The measurement of gait. Clinical Rehabilitation 2: 89–97
Butland RJ, Pang J, Gross ER, Woodcock AA, Geddes DM 1981 Two, six and twelve minute walks compared. Thorax 36(3): 225
Butler P, Engelbrecht M, Major RE, Tait JH, Stallard JS, Patrick JH 1984 Physiological cost index of walking for normal children and its use as an indicator of physical handicap. Developmental Medicine and Child Neurology 26: 607–612

Clarkson BH 1983 Absorbent paper for recording foot placement during gait. Physical Therapy 63(3) March: 345–346
Craik R, Oatis C 1985 Gait assessment in the clinic: issues and approaches. In: Rothstein J (Ed) Measurement in Physical Therapy. Churchill Livingstone, New York, Ch 6
Davis RB 1997 Reflections on clinical gait analysis. Journal of Electromyography 7(4): 251–257
Eastlack ME, Arvidson J, Synder-Mackler L, Danoff JV, McGarvey CL 1991 Inter-rater reliability of videotaped

observational gait-analysis assessments. Physical 7Therapy 71 (6): 465–472

Goodkin R, Diller L 1973 Reliability among physical therapists in diagnosis and treatment of gait deviations in hemiplegics. Perceptual and Motor Skills 37: 727–734

Gulmans VAM, van Veldhoven, NHMJ, deMeer K, Helders PJM 1996 The six-minute walking test in children with cystic fibrosis: Reliability and validity. Pediatric Pulmonology 22(2): 85–89

Hughes KA, Bell F 1994 Visual assessment of hemiplegic gait following stroke — Pilot study. Archives of Physical Medicine Rehabilitation 75(10): 1100–1107

Inman VT, Ralston HJ, Todd F 1981 Human Walking. Williams and Wilkins, Baltimore, MD

Kinsman R 1986 Video assessment of the Parkinson patient. Physiotherapy 72(8): 386–389

Kippen SC 1993 A preliminary assessment of recording the physical dimensions of an inked footprint. Journal British Podiatric Medicine. May: 74–80

Kopf A, Pawelka S, Kranzl A 1998 Clinical gait analysis—methods, limitations, and indications. Acta Medica Austriaca 25(1): 27–32

Krebs DE, Edelstein JE, Fishman S 1985 Reliability of observational kinematic gait analysis. Physical Therapy 65(7) July: 1027–1033

Law HT, Minns RA 1989 Measurement of the spatial and temporal parameters of gait. Physiotherapy 75(2): 81–84

Lord SE, Halligan PW, Wade DT 1998 Visual gait analysis: the development of a clinical assessment and scale. Clinical Rehabilitation 12: 107–119

Little N 1981 Gait Analysis: a survey of current methods. Physiotherapy 67(11): 334–337

Lower Limb Orthotics 1981 New York University Postgraduate Medical School. Prosthetics and Orthotics

McGregor J 1981 Evaluation of patient performance using long term ambulatory monitoring technique in domestic environment. Physiotherapy 67(2): 30

McNicol MF, McHardy R, Chalmers J 1980 Exercise testing before and after hip arthroplasty. Journal of Bone and Joint Surgery 62B(3): 326–331

McNicol MF, Uprichard H, Mitchell GP 1981 Exercise testing after the chiari pelvic osteotomy. Journal of Bone and Joint Surgery 63B(1): 48–52

Mendeiros J 1984 Automated measurement systems for clinical motion analysis. Physical Therapy 64(12): 1846–1850

Mulder T, Nienhuis B, Pauwels J 1998 Clinical gait analysis in a rehabilitation context. Clinical Rehabilitation 12(2): 99–106

Nene AV 1993 Physiological cost index of walking in able-bodied adolescents and adults. Clinical Rehabilitation 7: 319–326

Patla AE, Proctor J, Morson B 1987 Observations on aspects of visual gait assessment: a questionnaire study. Physiotherapy Canada 39(5): 311–316

Perry J 1992 Gait analysis: Normal and Pathological Function. Slack Inc., New Jersey,. USA

Rancho Los Amigos Medical Center 1989 Observational Gait Analysis Handbook. Los Amigos Research and Education Institute, Dorney, CA

Reimers J 1972 A scoring system for the evaluation of ambulation in cerebral palsy patients. Developmental Medicine and Child Neurology 14: 332–335

Robinson JL, Smidt GL 1981 Quantitative gait evaluation in the clinic. Physical Therapy 61(3): 351–353

Rose GK 1983 Clinical gait assessment: a personal view. Journal of Medical Engineering and Technology 7: 273–279

Rothstein J 1985 Measurement in Physical Therapy. Churchill Livingstone, New York

Rowe PJ, Nicol AC, Kelly IG 1989 Flexible goniometer computer system for the assessment of hip function. Clinical Biomechanics 4(2): 68–72

Shores M 1980 Footprint analysis in gait documentation. Physical Therapy 60(9): 1163–1167

Silvino N, Evanski PM, Waugh TR 1980 The Harris and Beath footprinting mat: diagnostic validity and clinical use. Clinical Orthopaedics and Related Research 151: 265–269

Singh SJ 1992 The use of field walking tests for assessment of functional capacity in patients with chronic airways obstruction. Physiotherapy 78(2): 102–104

Singh SJ, Morgan MDL, Scott S, Walters D, Hardman AE 1992 Development of a shuttle walking test of disability in patients with chronic airways obstruction. Thorax 47(12): 1019–1024

Smith A 1993 Variability in human locomotion: are repeat trials necessary? Australian Journal of Physiotherapy 39(2): 115–123

SMS Health Care Ltd 1998 Manufacturer's information. GAITRite Walkway System. SMS Health Care Ltd Harlow, Essex

Steadman J, Archer A, Jackson H et al 1997a Impairment and walking disability following stroke: a multi-centre study. Clinical Rehabilitation 11(1): 81–89

Steadman J, Archer A, Jackson H et al 1997b Is there a link between patients perception of their walking and objective walking performance following stroke? Age and Ageing 26 (Suppl 1): 26

Stuberg WA, Colerick VL, Blanke DJ, Bruce W 1988 Comparison of a clinical gait-analysis method using videography and temporal-distance measures with 16 mm cinematography. Physical Therapy 68(8): 1221–1225

Sutherland D, Olshen R, Cooper L, Woo S 1980 The development of mature gait. Journal of Bone and Joint Surgery 62A(3): 336–353

Volpon JB 1994 Footprint analysis during the growth period. Journal of Pediatric Orthopaedics 14: 83–85

Wade D, Wood V, Heller A, Maggs J, Langton Hewer R 1987 Walking after stroke. Scandinavian Journal of Rehabilitation Medicine 19: 25–30

Wade D 1992 Measurement in Neurological Rehabilitation. Oxford University Press, Oxford, UK

Wall JC 1991 Measurement of temporal gait parameters from videotape using a field counting technique. International Rehabilitation Research 14(4): 344–347

Wall JC, Ashburn A, Klenerman L 1981 Gait analysis in the assessment of functional performance before and after total hip replacement. Journal of Biomedical Engineering 3: 121–127

Wall JC, Crosbie J 1996 Accuracy and reliability of temporal gait measurement. Gait and Posture 4: 293–296

Wall JC, Crosbie J 1997 Temporal gait analysis using slow video and a personal computer. Physiotherapy 83(3): 109–115

Whittle M 1996a Clinical gait analysis: a review. Human Movement Science 15: 369–387

Whittle M 1996b Gait Analysis: an Introduction, 2nd edn. Butterworth–Heinemann, Oxford, pp 131–219

Winter DA 1987 The Biomechanics and Motor Control of Human Gait. University of Waterloo Press, Ontario, Ontario

Winter DA, Patla AE, Frank JS, Walt SE 1990 Biomechanical walking pattern changes in the fit and healthy elderly. Physical Therapy 70(6): 340–347

Wolfson L, Whipple R, Amerman P, Tobin J 1990 Gait assessment in the elderly: a gait abnormality rating scale and its relationship to falls. Journal of Gerontology 45(1): M12–M19

Worsfold C, Simpson JM 1996 The repeatability and acceptability of a stopwatch timed 3 metre walk among elderly in-patients. Society for Research in Rehabilitation, London

Yack HJ 1984 Techniques for clinical assessment of human movement. Physical Therapy 64(12): 1821–1829

9

Specific soft-tissue mobilization in the management of soft-tissue dysfunction

D. Hunter

Department of Physiotherapy and Occupational Therapy, Faculty of Health and Social Care, University of the West of England, Bristol, UK

Following injury, the ability of soft tissue to tolerate the demands of functional loading decreases. A major part of the management of soft-tissue dysfunction lies in promoting soft-tissue adaptation to restore the tissue's ability to cope with functional loading. Specific soft-tissue mobilization (SSTM) uses specific, graded and progressive application of force by the use of physiological, accessory or combined techniques either to promote collagen synthesis, orientation and bonding in the early stages of the healing process, or to promote changes in the viscoelastic response of the tissue in the later stages of healing. SSTM should be applied in combination with rehabilitation regimes to restore the kinetic control of the tissue. The principles of SSTM are reviewed with regard to the general principles of treating soft-tissue dysfunction and areas identified for further research in this field. *Manual Therapy* (1998) **3(1),** 2–11

INTRODUCTION

Until fairly recently, the majority of physio-therapy-based manual therapies have focused on assessment and treatment philosophies biased towards joint mechanics (Maitland 1991; Edwards 1992; Cyriax 1993). More recently, increasing attention has been given to management philosophies based on soft-tissue physiology and biomechanics aimed at reducing soft-tissue tightness, restoring soft-tissue mobility and correcting muscular imbalances (Butler

& Gifford 1989; Norris 1995; Richardson & Jull 1995; Shacklock 1995). Despite this recent trend towards soft-tissue-based philosophies, little emphasis has been given to the role that manual therapy has in the treatment of benign soft-tissue pathology, such as the inflammatory and degenerative lesions that occur following micro or macro trauma, with the result that treatment of these pathologies tends to be based on electrothermal rather than manual approaches. The notable exception has been Cyriax, who advocated the use of deep transverse frictions to 'break down' scar tissue and promoted collagen orientation during the healing process (Cyriax 1993). Although this approach is widely used and has a feasible biological hypothesis regarding the proposed mechanism of action, the evidence regarding the clinical effectiveness of deep transverse frictions has been negative (Walker 1984; Stratford et al 1989; Schwellnus & Mackintosh 1992; Pellecchia et al 1994). Paradoxically, despite the lack of research data supporting the effectiveness of deep transverse frictions, considerable evidence is accumulating to support the importance of carefully applied movement in restoring the tensile strength and functional biomechanical properties of healing tissue (Forrester et al 1970; Burroughs & Dahners 1990; Dahners & Padgett 1990; Karpakka et al 1990; Gomez et al 1991; Jarvinen & Lehto 1993; Muneta et al 1993). On the basis of this accumulating research evidence, the author proposed an assessment and treatment approach termed SSTM as an attempt to standardize a way of using manual therapy to treat benign soft-tissue pathology, and to offer a more sensitive and specific approach than the more traditionally used deep transverse frictions (Hunter 1994). SSTM uses graded and progressive applications of force matched as closely as possible to the stage of the healing process, in order to increase the tensile strength of the tissue and to restore the functional biomechanical properties of the soft tissue. This article describes the principles of SSTM in relation to the general principles of managing soft-tissue dysfunction.

GENERAL PRINCIPLES IN THE TREATMENT OF SOFT-TISSUE DYSFUNCTION

The soft tissues of the body are subjected to tensile, compressive and shear forces (Nordin & Frankel 1989). Following tissue overload, the ability of the soft tissue to tolerate force decreases, and therefore a major emphasis in the treatment process is to promote tissue adaptation to restore the tissue's ability to withstand the specific demands of functional loading. To achieve this successfully, the manual therapist must base treatment upon a detailed assessment process (Maitland 1991), specifically and progressively load the site of tissue dysfunction (Hunter 1994), and restore 'normal' kinetic control of the area (Norris 1995). In this article, three areas of the assessment and treatment of soft tissue dysfunction will receive specific attention:

1. Identification of the aetiology of injury and aggravating factors in relation to the soft tissue dysfunction
2. Identification of the site of tissue dysfunction and application of treatment to restore the tissue's biophysical properties in relation to specific functional demands
3. Specific progressive rehabilitation programmes to ensure adequate control of the affected area to reduce the risk of injury recurrence.

IDENTIFICATION OF THE AETIOLOGY OF INJURY AND AGGRAVATING FACTORS IN RELATION TO THE SOFT-TISSUE DYSFUNCTION

Soft-tissue dysfunction occurs when:

1. The load is excessive in relation to the mechanical properties of the tissue
2. The biomechanical properties of the tissue have decreased in relation to a 'normal load' (Leadbetter 1992)
3. Both 1 and 2 occur together.

Table 9.1 Factors to consider in determining the possible aetiology of soft-tissue dysfunction. See Caine et al (1996) for a more extensive analysis of this area.

Intrinsic factors Factors inherent in the person	Extrinsic factors Factors external to the person	Task-related factors Factors relating to task performance
Somatotype	Direct force results in either acute or insidious onset of injury. In sport the force may be legal or illegal	Technique
Age and gender		Preparation, e.g. warm up
Personality (e.g. risk takers)	Environmental factors, e.g. weather — temperature, humidity, wind; type of surface; altitude	Type of task
Posture and body mechanics, e.g. hypermobility, bone density, leg length, excessive pro- or supination, muscle imbalance — strength, power, endurance, control and flexibility, adverse neurodynamics, skill and coordination	Equipment, e.g. footwear. Is protective equipment worn? Is protective equipment worn correctly? Is the equipment the correct size and weight?	Adequate coaching or instruction Temporal factors — how long is the task performed for? How long are the rest periods? Intensity of the task
Poor rehabilitation from previous dysfunction	Social pressures	
Unsafe manipulation of physiology		Ergonomic considerations
Genetic predisposition		

Establishing the aetiology of soft-tissue dysfunction is important so that these factors can be corrected during the treatment process to reduce the risk of re-injury. However, many plausible aetiological theories lack substantive evidence in terms of causation because they are based on tests that have dubious validity and poor repeatability (McPoil & Cornwall 1996; Buckley & Hunt 1997). Establishing the validity and repeatability of all clinical tests should be a major research focus in future years in the appraisal of their clinical value.

Even when allowing for a lack of confidence in testing procedures, establishing a causative relationship is extremely conjectural bearing in mind the multi-factorial nature of the forces applied to the tissue and care should be used when interpreting a relationship as being causative (Meeuwisse 1994).

Allowing for these limitations, aetiological factors should be explored in relation to intrinsic, extrinsic, and task-related factors (Table 9.1). Watson (1997) provides an excellent review of this area.

As well as correcting possible aetiological factors, movement patterns that aggravate the current symptoms by loading the dysfunctional site beyond its mechanical capabilities should be controlled during the treatment process to avoid sabotaging any beneficial treatment effect. Taping or bracing is often useful to achieve this effect (Snyder-Mackler & Epler 1989).

IDENTIFICATION OF THE SITE OF TISSUE DYSFUNCTION AND APPLICATION OF TREATMENT TO RESTORE THE TISSUE'S BIOPHYSICAL PROPERTIES IN RELATION TO SPECIFIC FUNCTIONAL DEMANDS

Once the site of tissue dysfunction has been established through careful subjective and physical testing, progressive tensioning of the tissue is required to restore the mechanical properties to a level compatible with the potential imposed demands (Lehto & Jarvinen 1991; Muneta et al 1993). To do this successfully, tension is applied with respect to a treatment model based on current knowledge regarding soft-tissue biomechanics and the healing process of soft tissues.

BIOMECHANICAL PROPERTIES OF SOFT TISSUES

The tensile properties of soft tissues are com-monly investigated experimentally by applying a progressive tensile load to the tissue and measuring the resultant change in tissue length. This allows the investigator to plot either a load deformation curve, or if the tissue dimensions are taken into account, a stress–strain curve (Fig. 9.1).

The stress–strain curve is typically divided into four regions (Fig. 9.1). The main features relevant to the application of SSTM are as follows:

1. The slope in the linear portion of the curve (the elastic modulus) represents the tissue stiffness (Fig. 9.2) (Burstein & Wright 1994a). The stiffer the tissue, the steeper the slope and the more resistance experienced on tensioning the tissue, e.g. following chronic scar tissue formation. Historically, emphasis has been placed on using the ultimate failure point of the tissue to determine its biomechanical properties; however, the slope of the curve may be more informative with regards to the mechanical behaviour of the tissue *in vivo* as it represents the region of physiological loading (Butler et al 1984).

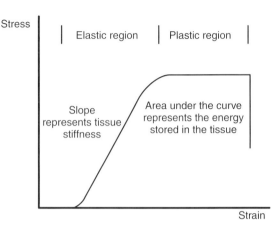

Figure 9.2 Stress–strain curve illustrating key areas of interest regarding the application of SSTM. SSTM may reduce tissue stiffness and, therefore, the inclination of the slope. This, in turn, affects the viscoelastic response of the tissue and its ability to store energy. Force applied into the plastic region results in permanent tissue elongation.

2. The area under the curve represents the energy stored in the tissue (Fig. 9.2) (Burstein & Wright 1994). This energy can be useful in improving efficiency as part of the stretch shorten cycle, i.e. eccentric to concentric muscle activity (Blanpied et al 1995; Fukashiro et al 1995; Keskula 1996), or it may be detrimental in terms of producing tendon pathology (Wilson & Goodship 1994). However, the greater the energy stored in the tissue, the greater the demands placed upon the tissue architecture. Following injury, the tissue architecture is less able to withstand the stress of tensile loading, hence the need to avoid excessive immobilization and to encourage early specific tissue loading to restore the tissue's ability to withstand and 'store' the applied energy (Akeson et al 1980; Woo et al 1987).

3. The stiffness of the tissue and the energy stored is influenced by the tissue's viscoelastic properties (Threlkeld 1992). Viscoelasticity is a property of soft tissues whereby the strain induced in the tissue is dependent on the rate of loading of the applied stress (Burstein & Wright 1994). It is thought to be due to biochemical interaction

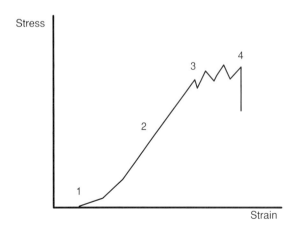

Figure 9.1 Stress–strain curve illustrating the four main informative regions of the curve. 1= toe region; 2= linear region; 3= fibre failure point; 4= ultimate failure point.

between the collagen fibres and the ground substance (Binkley 1989). In general, the faster the rate of loading, the stiffer the tissue becomes and the more energy is 'stored' in the tissue. This allows the tissue to withstand larger forces when the force is delivered more rapidly, a valuable attribute in tendons (Oakes 1994).

4. The stress–strain curve can be divided into elastic and plastic regions (Fig. 9.2). Loading the tissue within the elastic region results in a return to its original length once the load is removed. Loading the tissue within the plastic region results in permanent deformation of the tissue, which is therapeutically desirable when a decrease in tissue motion relates to the patient's symptoms.

5. Hysteresis is a phenomenon associated with energy loss exhibited by viscoelastic materials when they are subjected to loading and unloading cycles (Soderberg 1997). An elastic material demonstrates identical stress–strain curves during loading and unloading; however, with viscoelastic materials the curves of the two phases are not identical (Fig. 9.3). The area between the unloading and loading curves represents the energy that is lost due to mechanical damage to the tissue and from internal

friction (Burstein & Wright 1994b). Inducing hysteresis in the tissue helps to reduce tissue stiffness and restore the tissues' 'normal' mechanical response to loading (Garde 1988).

6. Creep is characterized by a continued deformation at a fixed load (Taylor et al 1990). The material continues to deflect until an equilibrium point is reached (Fig. 9.4). The clinical application of a constant low load over a prolonged period takes advantage of the creep response and is useful for increasing soft-tissue mobility (Carlstedt & Nordin 1989).

On the basis of the above principles it is possible to hypothesize that changes in the mechanical properties of soft tissue induced by SSTM may occur due to creep, plastic deformation and hysteresis, which alter the viscoelastic response and tissue architecture.

THE HEALING PROCESS OF SOFT TISSUES

Soft-tissue dysfunction usually arises from inflammatory or degenerative pathology. For a more extensive review see Woo & Buckwalter (1987).

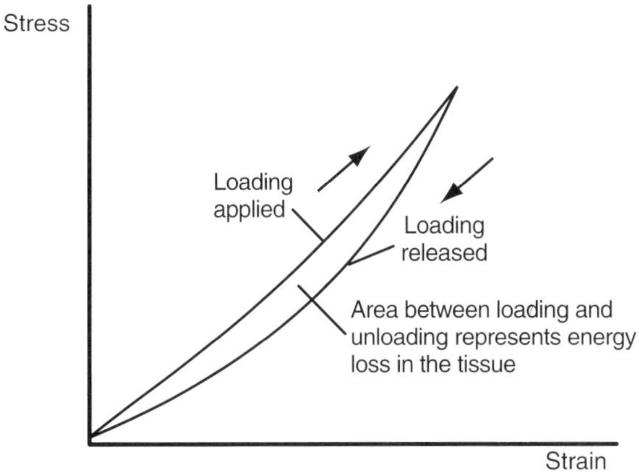

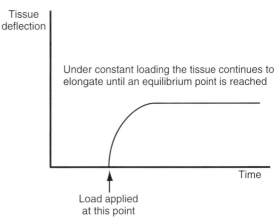

Figure 9.3 Hysteresis is a property exhibited by viscoelastic materials whereby energy loss occurs in the tissue during loading and unloading cycles. This energy loss is believed to occur due to structural damage and internal friction.

Figure 9.4 Creep occurs when a tissue that has been subjected to constant loading elongates until an equilibrium point is reached. The change in tissue length is of value if the decrease in motion is related to the patient's symptoms.

INFLAMMATORY PATHOLOGY

Following injury the tensile strength of the tissue decreases, and a major component of the healing process is to restore tensile strength to the damaged tissue. During the healing process the tensile strength of the tissue passes through three phases: the lag, regeneration and remodelling (Fig. 9.5). These phases are not clearly delineated in terms of time, and the length of each is influenced by many factors and is highly variable.

Lag phase

Typically the lag phase lasts between 4 and 6 days. During this time the inflammatory reaction prepares the wound for the regeneration phase (Barlow & Willoughby 1992). The wound is fragile, being stabilized by a weak fibrin bond, and tension applied during this time period may disrupt the fibrin and exacerbate the inflammatory response (Wahl et al 1989). Specific tension should not be applied to the site of tissue dysfunction during this time of vulnerability, and this should be a period of control with regard to the inflammatory reaction. The principles of rest, ice, compression, elevation and taping to restrict motion now appear to be valuable (Knight 1995). Ice may be more effective at this point if its use is based around the principle of preventing secondary hypoxia rather than the vasodilatation/constriction model commonly applied in physiotherapy (Knight 1995). Ultrasound may be useful during the lag phase (Webster et al 1978).

Regeneration phase

This is the period of the greatest increases in tensile strength due to the degree of collagen synthesis. The tendency for the formation of randomly orientated collagen fibres that restore structure but hinder function (Gomez et al 1991) can be reduced by careful tensioning of the healing tissue during the regeneration phase (Arem & Madden 1976). Specific tension may increase collagen synthesis, promote functional collagen alignment and increase collagen cross-

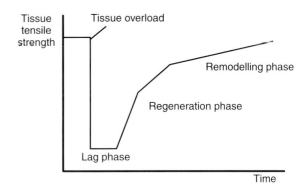

Figure 9.5 Hypothetical model of the three stages of the healing process in relation to the tensile strength of the healing tissue. (Modified from Hunter 1994, with permission.)

linkages so that they become more stable. This promotes a greater increase in tensile strength and reduces the time of the remodelling phase that follows (Currier & Nelson 1992).

Remodelling phase

The tensile strength of the tissue improves due to the formation of intra- and extramolecular cross-linkages between the collagen fibres (Currier & Nelson 1992). The tissue may become stiffer and less able to tolerate the demands of functional loading. SSTM may alter the mechanical properties of the tissue in terms of its viscoelastic response by promoting hysteresis, creep and plastic deformation.

In summary, SSTM has no role during the lag phase, but in the regeneration and remodelling phases it may be effective in re-orientating collagen fibres, increasing collagen number and affecting the viscoelastic response of the tissue. This may result in an earlier restoration of tensile strength in the tissue, and, therefore, an earlier return to 'normal' function (Fig. 9.6).

DEGENERATIVE PATHOLOGY

Evidence is accumulating that many 'inflammatory lesions', e.g. achilles tendinitis and patella

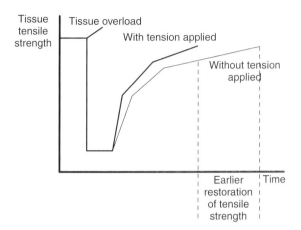

Figure 9.6 Hypothetical effect of specific and progressive SSTM during the regeneration and remodelling phases. Promotion of collagen synthesis, orientation and bonding may result in an earlier restoration of tensile strength to the tissue.

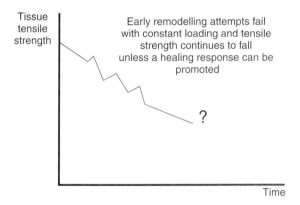

Figure 9.7 Hypothetical model of the effect of degenerative pathology on tissue tensile strength. The lack of research into degenerative pathology prevents the outcome of degenerative pathology from being depicted in this model.

tendinitis, may, in certain cases, be degenerative rather than inflammatory (Kannus 1997). Kannus & Jozsa (1991) suggest that degenerative tendon changes are evident in one third of the healthy urban population aged 35 years or more. In this degenerate state, hypoxic degenerative tendinopathy, mucoid degeneration, tendolipomatosis, calcifying tendinopathy or their combi-

nation may be found at biopsy (Kannus & Jozsa 1991). The absence of inflammation means that there is no stimulus for the normal healing response, and the application of SSTM in this case may produce an inflammatory response that initiates healing (Fig. 9.7). There is some evidence that eccentric training regimes to promote tendon remodelling may be of value in the treatment of degenerate tendon dysfunction (Stanish et al 1986); however, this approach has yet to be subjected to prospective, randomized studies to evaluate clinical effectiveness with regard to other treatment approaches.

SPECIFIC SOFT-TISSUE MOBILIZATION TECHNIQUES

The aim of SSTM varies depending on the stage of the healing process during which it is applied. Immediately following the lag phase the aim is to promote collagen synthesis, orientation and bond stability. In the later stages of the healing reaction, the aim is to alter the mechanical properties of the tissue with respect to its viscoelastic response to loading, based on the principles of hysteresis, creep and plastic deformation.

To apply tension to the specific site of tissue dysfunction, the author has suggested the following classification of techniques (Hunter 1994):

1. Physiological SSTM
2. Accessory SSTM
3. Combined SSTM.

Physiological specific soft-tissue mobilization

Physiological joint movement is used to apply tension to the specific site of tissue dysfunction. This is achieved by finding the correct sequence of physiological joint motion that relates to soft-tissue tension based on the degrees of freedom occurring at the joint or joints over which the soft tissue has an influence. For example, in a patient with dysfunction at the musculotendinous junction of the biceps femoris, combinations of hip flexion, medial rotation and adduction together with knee extension and medial tibial rotation

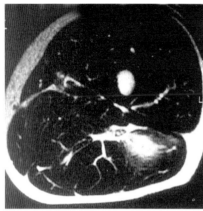

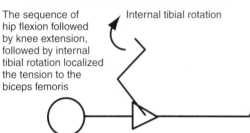

The sequence of hip flexion followed by knee extension, followed by internal tibial rotation localized the tension to the biceps femoris

Internal tibial rotation

Figure 9.8 T2 weighted MRI scan of a muscle tendon unit strain of the biceps femoris. This patient's symptoms were reproduced by the sequence of hip flexion with the knee flexed, followed by knee extension, followed by internal rotation of the tibia. Without tibial internal rotation the hip and knee sequence of physiological SSTM was relatively asymptomatic.

should be explored to locate the tension to the dysfunctional site (Fig. 9.8). The use of uniplanar physiological techniques that are commonly recommended in relation to 'stretching exercises' or assessing soft tissue 'length' fail to acknowledge that different parts of a soft tissue are tensioned by different combinations of joint motion. On this basis, there is no single physiological stretch for all parts of a soft tissue, only for some parts thereof. It is only when all areas of the soft tissue have been subjected to tension by varying combinations of physiological SSTM that a tissue can be claimed to have full physiological extensibility and clinical tensile strength. In assessing the correct sequence of physiological SSTM, the concept of the order effect is important, as the same physiological movements applied in a different order affects the perceived

location of stretch (Ayre et al 1996). This may relate to the fact that the muscle tendon unit does not behave homogeneously when under tension (Best 1993).

Careful attention should be paid to the shoulder and pelvic girdles in relation to tensioning associated tissues. Lack of stabilization at these sites results in a decreased ability to tension the more proximal aspect of the tissue; for example, when tensioning the rectus femoris with the sequence of either hip extension followed by knee flexion, or vice versa, the pelvis will tend to tilt anteriorly, which decreases the tension at the proximal attachment of the rectus femoris. Therefore, a posterior pelvic tilt is important during this procedure if the stretch is to be more localized in the proximal aspect of the tissue.

Provided no joint instability is evident, physiological SSTM is used to tension ligamentous tissue by applying the same principles as above. For example, inversion at various degrees of plantar flexion is used to tension the specific site of dysfunction in the anterior talofibular ligament (Fig. 9.9). Tensioning the ligament through the available joint range is important as different ligamentous fibres are tensioned at different degrees of joint motion. In certain areas, physiological SSTM can be made more specific by the addition of accessory joint motion after the tissue has been tensioned using physiological SSTM: for example, a posterior glide of the lateral malleolus following plantar flexion and inversion to further tension the anterior talofibular ligament, or an anterior glide of the humeral head after the physiological movements of abduction and medial rotation have been used to tension certain fibres in the infraspinatus (Fig. 9.10).

During the assessment of physiological SSTM, the range, quality and limiting factors are noted. Specific attention should be paid to the perceived area of sensation so that this can be related to a 'normal' pattern for that movement sequence. In certain areas of the body, physiological SSTM is unable to specifically tension the site of tissue dysfunction, for example in relation to the deeper muscles of the adductor region, and in these cases accessory SSTM is utilized to make the technique more specific.

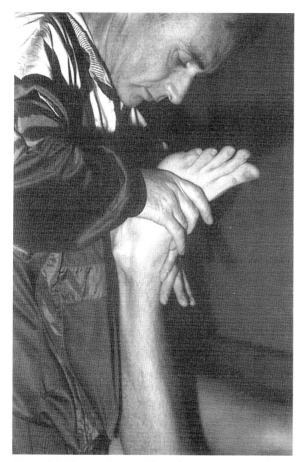

Figure 9.9 Plantar flexion followed by inversion tensions the anterior component of the lateral ligament of the ankle joint. The inversion stress should be applied through the range of plantar flexion that tensions the specific site of tissue dysfunction.

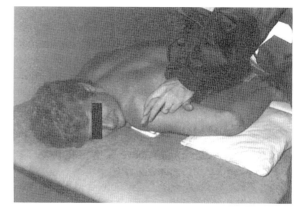

Figure 9.10 Physiological movements of glenohumeral abduction and medial rotation are applied to tension the site of dysfunction in the infraspinatus. An anterior glide of the humeral head may be used to make the tension more specific.

Deep transverse frictions

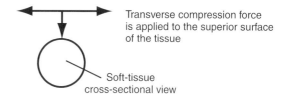

Transverse compression force is applied to the superior surface of the tissue

Soft-tissue cross-sectional view

Accessory SSTM

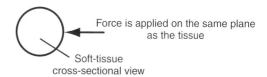

Force is applied on the same plane as the tissue

Soft-tissue cross-sectional view

Figure 9.11 Comparison between the method of force application for deep transverse frictions and accessory SSTM.

Accessory specific soft-tissue mobilization

Accessory SSTM is performed by applying direct pressure on the same tissue plane and at 90° to the site of soft-tissue dysfunction. Unlike deep transverse frictions that exert a compressive and transverse force on the superior surface of the tissue, accessory SSTM pushes against the tissue, displacing the tissue axis and resulting in increased longitudinal tension within the tissue (Fig. 9.11). The transverse pressure on the same plane as the tissue dysfunction allows the therapist to assess the range, quality and limiting factors of the tissue motion and to grade the application of force to the tissue's biomechanical capabilities in relation to the stage of the healing process. The palpatory information relating to the quality of tissue motion is richer with accessory SSTM in relation to deep transverse frictions, and, therefore, clinically more informative; however

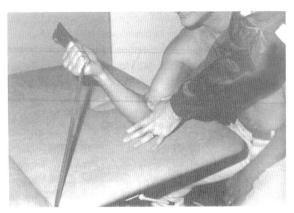

Figure 9.12 In the later stages of treating muscle–tendon unit dysfunction, accessory SSTM is applied while the tissue undergoes isometric, concentric or eccentric muscle activity. Here the bicipital aponeurosis is treated with accessory SSTM while the patient performs a concentric biceps contraction.

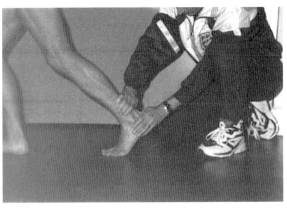

Figure 9.13 Combined SSTM applied to the Achilles tendon during functional weight-bearing activity.

differences in these are clinical effectiveness between the two approaches.

Usually, accessory SSTM is applied with the tissue relaxed; however, in the later stages of the treatment of musculotendinous dysfunction, accessory SSTM is used in combination with isometric, concentric or eccentric muscle activity to localize the tension more specifically to the site of tissue dysfunction (Fig. 9.12).

Combined specific soft-tissue mobilization

The specific site of soft-tissue dysfunction is placed under tension by the use of physiological SSTM and then accessory SSTM techniques are used to increase the specificity of the tension. Because combined SSTM exerts the most tension at the site of dysfunction, it is generally used towards the later stages of the treatment process, and also often with functional or weight-bearing loading (Fig. 9.13).

TECHNIQUE APPLICATION

The difficulty in applying force to dysfunctional tissue lies in establishing how much force is required to promote adaptation but not failure

(Leibovic & McDowell 1994). The lack of research in this area means that SSTM application is based on experience rather than formula, under the guidance of severity, irritability and underlying pathology, as well as subjective and physical retesting (Maitland 1991). The variables that must be considered are as follows.

Type of force

An oscillatory force is recommended in the early stages of the healing process (from approximately days 6 to 14 for a mild to moderate lesion) to facilitate dispersal of inflammatory exudate and gently tension the lesion. After this time period a sustained force with slow oscillation into resistance is recommended to promote hysteresis, creep and plastic deformation.

Grade of force

In the early stages of the healing process an oscillatory movement, equivalent to a Grade 2 (Maitland 1991), is recommended. Beyond the early stages (day 6–14) a sustained technique with slow oscillation into resistance, equivalent to a Grade 4 (Maitland 1991) is recommended. In both cases the therapist aims to apply the force

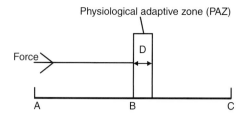

Physiological adaptive zone (PAZ)

A to C = 'Normal' range of accessory or physiological soft tissue motion.

A to B = Decreased soft tissue motion due to pathology.

Force applied with the correct grade enters the zone of physiological adaptation (D) promoting tissue adaption and gradual movement of the PAZ to the right.

Force graded to less than the PAZ fails to achieve a treatment effect.

Force graded beyond the PAZ produces pathological rather than physiological adaptation.

Figure 9.14 Diagrammatic representation of the zone of physiological adaptation with regards to grading SSTM force application.

with the correct grade to promote physiological but not pathological adaptation (Fig. 9.14).

Direction of application

The tissue response to movement should be assessed in all directions, and treatment applied on the basis of the direction of motion that presents the most symptomatic response, comparable sign or the most beneficial changes in terms of subjective and physical re-testing.

Time of application

The absence of research evidence regarding the correct time for force application means that the therapist must select this parameter on the basis of tissue irritability, degree of tissue stiffness and subjective and physical changes. As a general rule, the author applies each force for between 30 and 60 seconds, with the number of repetitions of this force being guided by physical and subjective changes. The patient must regularly tension the area between treatment sessions and the author suggests a frequency of every 2 waking hours to patients.

Extensive research is needed to provide more objective data regarding the parameters of force application mentioned above.

SPECIFIC PROGRESSIVE REHABILITATION PROGRAMMES TO ENSURE ADEQUATE CONTROL OF THE AFFECTED AREA TO REDUCE THE RISK OF INJURY RECURRENCE

The mechanical model presented above focuses on the primary site of tissue dysfunction. The changes facilitated by SSTM are only successful in restoring 'normal' function if the tissue functions within the control of a kinetic environment which matches the imposed functional demands (Norris 1995). Specific and progressive rehabilitation programmes should proceed hand in hand with SSTM, to restore parameters relating to muscle control, proprioception, coordination, fitness and psychosocial factors.

CLINICAL EXAMPLE OF SPECIFIC SOFT-TISSUE MOBILIZATION IN THE TREATMENT OF ‘TENNIS ELBOW’

The pathology of tennis elbow is commonly multi-factorial (Nirschl 1986; Yaxley & Jull 1993). However, dysfunction of extensor carpi radialis brevis (ECRB) is proposed as a common mechanism of pain production in this multi-factorial model (Stoeckart et al 1989). The principles of SSTM applied to the treatment of ECRB dysfunction are illustrated as follows.

Physiological specific soft-tissue mobilization

Combinations of forearm pronation, wrist flexion, ulna deviation and individual finger flexion with the elbow in extension should be explored. The order effect of finger flexion followed by wrist flexion, and vice versa, should be evaluated to establish the most symptomatic pattern.

Physiological SSTM can be made more specific by direct pressure to the head of the third metacarpal. This accessory movement may localize the stretch more specifically to the ECRB (Fig. 9.15).

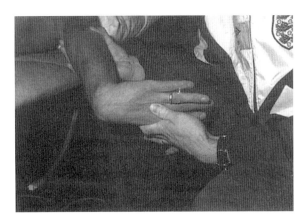

Figure 9.15 Physiological movements of elbow extension, forearm pronation, wrist flexion and ulnar deviation are used to localize the tension in the ECRB. Pressure applied to the third metacarpal may increase the specificity of the technique.

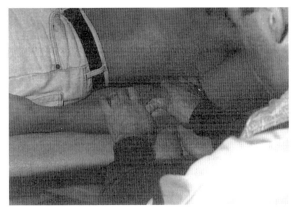

Figure 9.16 Accessory SSTM is applied on the same plane as the tissue dysfunction in the ECRB.

Accessory specific soft-tissue mobilization

With the wrist and fingers in neutral, the accessory motion of the tissue at the site of dysfunction is established; note range, quality and limiting factors (Fig. 9.16).

Combined specific soft-tissue mobilization

The correct sequence of physiological SSTM is applied followed by accessory SSTM at the site of tissue dysfunction. As treatment progresses, resistance by means of elastic bands or tubing is incorporated into the treatment programme (Fig. 9.17).

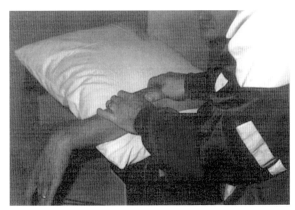

Figure 9.17 Combined SSTM is applied to localize the force to the site of tissue dysfunction. From this position resisted exercises are used to facilitate the tissue's ability to withstand the demands of functional loading. Note: the elastic tubing applied to the third finger.

CONCLUSION

An approach to the treatment of benign soft-tissue dysfunction has been presented. Although the application of specific, graded and progressive force to influence the healing process and mechanical properties of soft tissue appears to be based on sound biophysical principles, much of the supporting evidence is drawn from *in vitro* rather than *in vivo* data, and from animal rather than human tissue. Empirically, SSTM has important clinical value in the treatment of soft-tissue dysfunction, but empiricism deservedly has little credibility in the scientific environment in which practice takes place. It is the author's hope that this article is not seen just as a model on which to base treatment, but as an enticement to encourage discussion and research into the clinical value of manual therapy applied to soft-tissue dysfunction so that research into this area can extend beyond its current level of infancy.

REFERENCES

Akeson WH, Amiel D, Woo SL-Y 1980 Immobility effects on synovial joints. The pathomechanics of joint contracture. Biorheology 17: 95–110

Arem AJ, Madden JW 1976 Effects of stress on healing wounds: 1. Intermittent noncyclical tension. Journal of Surgical Research 20: 93–102

Ayre K, Jowett C, Hunter G 1996 The effects of different passive hamstring stretches on the perceived areas of stretch. BSc unpublished thesis, University of West of England, Bristol

Barlow Y, Willoughby J 1992 Pathophysiology of soft tissue repair. British Medical Bulletin 48(3): 698–711

Best TM 1993 A biomechanical study of skeletal muscle strain injuries. PhD unpublished thesis, Duke University, USA

Binkley J 1989 Overview of ligament and tendon structure and mechanics: implications for clinical practice. Physiotherapy Canada 41(1): 24–30

Blanpied PB, Levins JA, Murphy E 1995 The effects of different stretch velocities on average force of the shortening phase in the stretch shorten cycle. Journal of Orthopaedic and Sports Physical Therapy 21(6): 345–353

Buckley ER, Hunt DV 1997 Reliability of clinical measurement of subtalar joint movement. Foot and Ankle International 18(4): 229–232

Burroughs P, Dahners LE 1990 The effect of enforced exercise on the healing of ligament injuries. American Journal of Sports Medicine 18: 376–378

Burstein AH, Wright TM 1994 Orthopaedic Biomechanics. Williams & Wilkins, Baltimore, pp97–129

Butler D, Gifford L 1989 The concept of adverse mechanical tension in the nervous system. Physiotherapy 75(11): 622–636

Butler DL, Grood ES, Noyes FR, Zernicke RG, Barckett K 1984 The effects of structure and strain measurement technique on the material properties of young human tendons and fascia. Journal of Biomechanics 17: 579–596

Caine DJ, Caine CG, Linder KJ 1996 Epidemiology of Sports Injuries. Human Kinetics, Illinois

Carlstedt CA, Nordin M 1989 Biomechanics of tendons and ligaments. In: Nordin M, Frankel VH (eds) Basic Biomechanics of the Musculo-Skeletal System, 2nd edn. Lea & Febiger, Philadelphia, pp65–67

Currier DP, Nelson RM 1992 Dynamics of Human Biologic Tissues. FA Davis, Philadelphia

Cyriax J 1993 Cyriax's Illustrated Manual of Orthopaedic Medicine, 2nd edn. Butterworth–Heinemann, Edinburgh, pp19–23

Dahners LE, Padgett I 1990 The effect of joint motion on collagen organisation in healing ligaments. Transcriptions of Orthopaedic Research Society 15: 511

Edwards BC 1992 Manual of Combined Movements. Churchill Livingstone, Edinburgh

Forrester JC, Zenefeldt BH, Hayes TL, Hunt TK 1970 Wolff's law in relation to the healing skin wound. The Journal of Trauma 10(9): 770–779

Fukashiro S, Komi PV, Jarvinen M, Miyashita 1995 In vivo achilles tendon loading during jumping in humans. European Journal of Applied Physiology and Occupational Physiology 71: 453–458

Garde RE 1988 Cervical traction: the neurophysiology of lordosis and the rheological characteristics of cervical curve rehabilitation. In: Harrison DD (ed). Chiropractic: The Physics of Spinal Correction. Sunnyvale CA, pp535–659

Gomez MA, Woo SL-Y, Amiel D, Harwood F 1991 The effects of increased tension on healing medial collateral ligaments. American Journal of Sports Medicine 19: 347–354

Hunter G 1994 Specific soft tissue mobilisation in the treatment of soft tissue lesions. Physiotherapy 80(1): 15–21

Jarvinen MJ, Lehto MUK 1993 The effects of early mobilisation and immobilisation on the healing process following muscle injuries. Sports Medicine 15(2): 78–89

Kannus P 1997 Tendon pathology: basic science and clinical applications. Sports Exercise and Injury 3: 62–75

Kannus P, Jozsa L 1991 Histopathological changes preceding spontaneous rupture of a tendon. A controlled study of 891 patients. Journal of Bone and Joint Surgery (Am) 73: 1507–1525

Karpakka J, Vaananen K, Virtanen P, Savolainen, Orava S, Takai TES 1990 The effects of remobilisation and exercise in collagen biosynthesis in rat tendon. Acta Physiologica Scandinavica 139: 139–145

Keskula DR 1996 Clinical implications of eccentric exercise in sports medicine. Journal of Sports Rehabilitation 5: 321–329

Knight K 1995 Cryotherapy in Sports Medicine. Human Kinetics, Champaign, USA, pp85–98

Leadbetter WB 1992 Cell-matrix response in tendon injury. Clinics in Sports Medicine 11: 533–578

Lehto M, Jarvinen M 1991 Muscle injuries healing and treatment. Annals Chirurgiae et Gynaecologiae 80: 102–109

Leibovic SJ, McDowell CL 1994 Repair and healing of flexor tendons in the hand. Current Opinion in Orthopaedics 5: 81–86

Maitland G 1991 Peripheral Manipulation. Butterworth–Heinemann, London, pp13–46

McPoil TG, Cornwall MW 1996 The relationship between static lower extremity measurements and rearfoot motion during walking. Journal of Orthopaedic and Sports Physical Therapy 24(5): 309–314

Meeuwisse WH 1994 Assessing causation in sports injury: a multifactorial model. Clinical Journal of Sports Medicine 4: 166–170

Muneta T, Lewis J, Stewart N 1993 Effects of controlled load on graft healing: auto vs allograft. Transcriptions of the Orthopaedic Research Society 18: 4

Nirschl R 1986 Soft tissue injuries about the elbow. Clinics in Sports Medicine 5(4): 637–652

Nordin M, Frankel V 1989 Basic Biomechanics of the Musculo-Skeletal System, 2nd edn. Lea & Febiger, London, pp9–16

Norris CM 1995 Spinal stabilisation — muscle imbalance and the low back. Physiotherapy 81(3): 127–138

Oakes B 1994 Tendon-ligament basic science. In: Harries M, Williams C, Stanish WD, Micheli L J (eds) Oxford Book of Sports Medicine. Oxford University Press, New York, pp. 493–511

Pellecchia GL, Hamel H, Behnke P 1994 Treatment of infrapatellar tendinitis: a combination of modalities and transverse friction massage versus iontophoresis. Journal of Sports Rehabilitation 3: 135–145

Richardson C, Jull G 1995 Muscle control – pain control. What exercises would you prescribe? Manual Therapy 1: 2–10

Schwellnus MP, Mackintosh LJ 1992 Deep transverse frictions in the treatment of iliotibial band friction syndrome in athletes: a clinical trial. Physiotherapy 78: 564–568

Shacklock M 1995 Neurodynamics. Physiotherapy 81(1): 9–16

Snyder-Mackler L, Epler M 1989 Effect of standard and aircast tennis elbow bands on integrated electromyography of forearm extensor musculature proximal to the bands. American Journal of Sports Medicine 17(2): 278–281

Soderberg GL 1997 Kinesiology: application to pathological motion, 2nd edn. Williams & Wilkins, Baltimore, p. 107

Stanish WD, Rubinovich RM, Curwin S 1986 Eccentric exercise in chronic tendinitis. Clinical Orthopaedics 208: 65–68

Stoeckart R, Vleeming A, Snijders C J 1989 Anatomy of the extensor carpi radialis brevis muscle related to tennis elbow. Clinical Biomechanics 4(2): 210–212

Stratford PW, Levy DR, Gauldie S, Miseferi D, Levy K 1989 The evaluation of phonophoresis and friction massage as treatments for extensor carpi radialis tendinitis: a randomised controlled trial. Physiotherapy Canada 41: 93–99

Taylor DC, Dalton JD, Seaber AV, Garrett WE 1990 Viscoelastic properties of muscle tendon units: the biomechanical effects of stretching. American Journal of Sports Medicine 18(3): 300–309

Threlkeld AJ 1992 The effects of manual therapy on connective tissue. Physical Therapy 72(12): 893–902

Wahl SM, Wong H, McCartney-Francis N 1989 Role of growth factors in inflammation and repair. Journal of Cell Biochemistry 40: 343–351

Walker JM 1984 Deep transverse frictions in ligament healing. Journal of Orthopaedic and Sports Physical Therapy 6(2): 89–94

Watson AWS 1997 Sports injuries: incidence, causes, prevention. Physical Therapy Review 2: 135–151

Webster D, Pond JB, Dyson M, Harvey W 1978 The role of ultrasound induced cavitation on the in vitro stimulation of protein synthesis in human fibroblasts by ultrasound. Ultrasound in Medicine and Biology 4: 343–345

Wilson AM, Goodship AE 1994 Exercise induced hyperthermia as a possible mechanism for tendon degeneration. Journal of Biomechanics 27: 899–905

Woo SL-Y, Gomez MA, Sites TJ, Newton PO 1987 The biomechanical and morphological changes in the medial collateral ligament of the rabbit after immobilisation and remobilisation. Journal of Bone and Joint Surgery 69A(8): 1200–1211

Woo SL-Y, Buckwalter JA (eds) 1987 Injury and repair of the musculo-skeletal soft tissues. American Academy of Orthopaedic Surgeons, Illinois

Yaxley G, Jull G 1993 Adverse tension in the neural system. A preliminary study in patients with tennis elbow. Australian Journal of Physiotherapy 39(1): 15–22

POSTSCRIPT

With the passage of time and the application of critical thought, the hypotheses and theories used in clinical reasoning are developed, adapted and sometimes rejected. In this regard the arguments posed in the above article on the principles of SSTM have developed, particularly in the area of plausible mechanisms of action and in the generation of evidence to support the effectiveness of SSTM. These developments have resulted in a broader model of potential therapeutic action, which can be used to facilitate clinical reasoning and to formulate research questions. These developments are discussed in this brief reflection on the paper.

The key message in the above article was that graded application of force to a site of soft-tissue dysfunction was thought to produce adaptation in the mechanical properties of a tissue, thus enabling it to withstand the mechanical demands of function. This assertion was based on evidence substantiating a link between tissue mechanics and function. While this model has a good level of scientific support, it offers a narrow view of how the body potentially adapts to SSTM. Also, tissue adaptation takes time and hence the apparent rapid functional adaptation that may occur with some treatments can be difficult to justify with this model. A further limitation is that dysfunction may occur when the mechanical properties of a tissue are optimal.

Due to these limitations a broader model was required to explain the potential therapeutic effects of SSTM, one which acknowledged the mechanical link to dysfunction but also incorporated other potential models of action. In this regard the author has found the model described by Lederman (1997) particularly useful.

Lederman's (1997) model of manual therapy includes local, neurological and psychophysiological effects. Local effects take place local to the site of therapeutic force application and are suggested to be changes in tissue mechanics, influences on healing and degenerative processes and pressure changes. The mechanical model of SSTM fits into this category. The neurological and psychophysiological effects were not considered in the above article and yet they offer alternative plausible modes of action, particularly with regard to the management of chronic soft-tissue dysfunction. The neurological effects relate to pain modulation and reflex inhibition effects, which generate an interesting hypothesis with regard to the desensitization of chronic scar tissue and the peripheral modulation of central sensitivity. The psychophysiological effects relate to the autonomic and higher centre changes and the effects of manual therapy on these parameters. Extending the potential therapeutic effects of SSTM in this way provides opportunities for developing the clinical reasoning of the concept as well as generating ideas for further research.

In terms of the efficacy of SSTM, a randomized clinical trial was conducted into the management of plantar fascia dysfunction with SSTM (Jackson et al 2000). The results indicated a statistically significant improvement with SSTM over the use of ultrasound and control, but the low power of these studies restricts the level of therapeutic claims that can be made from this study. Further studies are currently underway to evaluate the effectiveness of SSTM.

REFERENCES

Jackson T, Hunter G, Swinkles A 2000 The effects of specific soft tissue mobilisation on the functional foot index score in patients with plantar fasciitis, unpublished MSc. thesis, University of the West of England, Bristol

Lederman E 1997 Fundamentals of Manual Therapy: Physiology, Neurology and Psychology, , Churchill Livingstone, Edinburgh pp1–4

10

Peripheral mobilizations with movement

Linda Exelby

Physiotherapy Department, Pinehill Hospital, North Herts, UK

The use of mobilizations with movement (MWM) for peripheral joints has been developed by Mulligan. A mobilization is applied parallel or at right angles to the restricted joint movement. If the applied mobilization achieves immediate improvement in the functional movement and abolishes the pain, the treatment involves sustaining the mobilization while the patient performs the active movement repetitively. On re-assessment of the joint function, the movement should remain improved without the mobilization. Theories as to why these techniques provide rapid improvement in pain-free range are proposed, and the general principles of examination and treatment are outlined. Specific clinical examples demonstrate how MWM can be used in isolation or integrated with other manual approaches to improve the quality of joint intraarticular gliding and neurodynamics and the facilitation of correct muscle recruitment.
Manual Therapy (1996) **1/1,** 118–126

INTRODUCTION

The use of Brian Mulligan's treatment approach of combining passive mobilizations with active movement in the management of musculoskeletal dysfunction has become widespread among manual physiotherapists in recent years. These techniques were pioneered by Mulligan in New Zealand in the 1970s. Mulligan incorporated Kaltenborn's (1989) principles of passive mobilization in this approach. The combination of an active movement with simultaneous passive accessory mobilizations directed along the zygapophyseal joint planes was used initially in the cervical spine. The techniques, performed in the weight-bearing position, were later found to be equally effective when treating other areas of the spine. They are thought to achieve painless movement by restoring the reduced accessory glide.

Similar principles can be applied to the treatment of peripheral musculoskeletal disorders and are termed MWM (Mulligan 1993, 1995). In essence, the limited painful physiological movement is performed actively while the therapist applies a sustained accessory glide at right angles or parallel to the joint. The aim is to restore a restricted, painful movement to a pain-free and full range state. These principles apply not only to painful active joint movements but may be equally effective when the presenting problem is pain on an isometric contraction of muscle around a joint. The treatment of choice would be a glide to the joint that allows a pain-free isometric contraction. The latter was found to be particularly useful in the treatment of tennis elbow when the contraction of the wrist extensor muscles was painful (Mulligan 1995; Vicenzino & Wright 1995).

This article proposes possible reasons for the rapid increase in pain-free movement, outlines the principles of treatment and illustrates via clinical examples how MWMs can be successfully utilized in the peripheral joints.

PROPOSED MECHANISMS

Mulligan (1995) proposed that a minor positional fault of the joint may occur following an injury or strain, resulting in movement restrictions or pain. Lewit (1985) has shown that reduced joint mobility can often be a result of a 'mechanical block' from inert structures within a joint. Joint afferent discharge and optimal muscle recruitment are closely linked (Stokes & Young 1984; Schaible & Grubb 1993). Joint movement can be reduced as a result of reflex muscle splinting (Lewit 1985; Schaible & Grubb 1993; Taylor et al 1994), which prevents further damage and reduces nociceptor discharge from the joint by holding it in the midrange position. It is suggested that treatment directed at the joint will have an effect on muscle activity and vice versa. Experiments carried out by Thabe (1986), Taylor et al (1994) and Murphy et al

(1995) using electromyography demonstrated that joint mobilization and manipulation had a reflex effect on the activity of segmental muscles. Baxendale & Ferrell (1981) and Lundberg et al (1978) have shown that end-range passive movements have a reflex inhibitory effect on the muscle acting over the joint. Gerrard and Matyas (1980), on the other hand, were unable to demonstrate any changes in muscle activity with gentle mobilization techniques performed in the resistance-free part of the range. This seems to indicate that to affect muscle reflexly via joint afferents the mobilization technique must be performed into resistance. However, to achieve the desired effect on muscle the mobilization must be performed into resistance without excessive pain, which would lead to an adverse effect on the segmental muscle (Cobb et al 1975). This can be demonstrated clinically when a mobilization performed too strongly results in protective muscle spasm.

MWMs provide a passive pain-free end-range corrective joint glide with an active movement. The combination of joint mobilization with active movement may be responsible for the rapid return of pain-free movement.

PRINCIPLES OF TREATMENT

Human joint surfaces are not fully congruent and physiological movements occur as a combination of a rotation and a glide (Williams 1995). The Kaltenborn and Mulligan concepts place particular emphasis on restoration of the glide component of joint movement to facilitate full pain-free range of movement. The various glides used with MWMs can be determined by applying Kaltenborn's conceptual model (1989):

CONVEX/CONCAVE RULE

The direction of decreased joint gliding in a hypomobile joint, and thus appropriate treatment, can be deduced by this rule. When the convex joint partner moves, the glide occurs in the opposite direction (Fig. 10.1); for example with shoulder abduction, a longitudinal caudad glide of the humerus occurs. With movement of a concave joint partner, the glide occurs in the same direction (Fig. 10.2); for example with knee flexion in non-weight-bearing, there is an anteroposterior (AP) glide of the tibia on the femur.

TREATMENT PLANE RULE

A treatment plane passes through the joint and lies at a right angle to a concave joint partner (Fig. 10.3). Treatment is always applied parallel to this treatment plane. Hinge joints often respond particularly well to this glide, and this may be a first treatment choice (Mulligan 1995).

In summary the mobilization or glide can be applied to a joint in two ways: (i) at right angles to the joint movement, e.g. a medial or lateral glide on the tibia when improving flexion and extension (Fig. 10.4). (ii) the appropriate glide can be determined by applying the concave convex rule, e.g. an AP glide on the tibia when improving knee flexion (Fig. 10.5).

If applying the above principles does not provide sufficient improvement, a more recent development is to apply a sustained rotation to the moving joint partner. The conjunct rotation normally accompanying the physiological active movement being treated may be the initial choice of technique.

When pain with movement occurs in the carpal or tarsal bone regions, this pain can often be eliminated by gliding one bone relative to another and combining this with the painful movement. With joint movements that involve adjacent long bones, such as at the wrist (radius and ulna), the ankle (tibia and fibula), the metatarsals and the metacarpals, it is often necessary to glide one long bone relative to the other to achieve pain-free movement.

EXAMINATION

The clinical examination of the musculoskeletal dysfunction aims to establish the diagnosis and determine the underlying causative factors of the patient's symptoms so that the appropriate treatment can be implemented. It is essential to identify and analyse both the movement

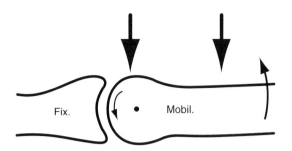

Figure 10.1 When the convex joint partner moves the glide occurs in the opposite direction. (Reproduced with kind permission from *Physiotherapy* 1995 81(12): 726–729.)

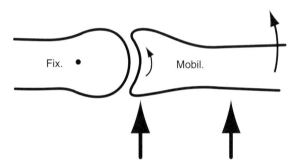

Figure 10.2 When the concave joint partner moves the glide occurs in the same direction. (Reproduced with kind permission from *Physiotherapy* 1995 81(12): 726–729.)

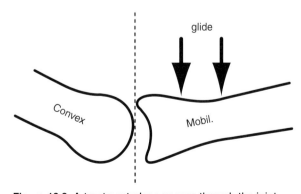

Figure 10.3 A treatment plane passes through the joint and lies at 90°to a concave joint partner. (Reproduced with kind permission from *Physiotherapy* 1995 81(12): 726–729).

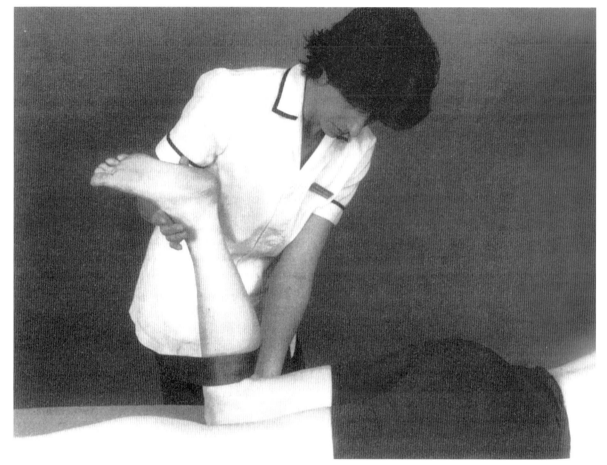

Figure 10.4 Lateral glide on tibia with active flexion. (Reproduced with kind permission from *Physiotherapy* 1995 81(12): 726–729.)

that precipitated the injury and functional activities that continue to exacerbate the symptoms. A knowledge of normal anatomy and biomechanics is essential so that abnormalities can be identified. Active and passive physiological movements and accessory glides are performed so that their contribution to the movement dysfunction and symptoms can be analysed. For example, if a patient has a painful limitation of wrist extension, the passive physiological and accessory components of radiocarpal and midcarpal extension should be assessed as well as the quality of the intercarpal accessory gliding. Taking the Kaltenborn (1989) concave/convex concept into consideration, if the radiocarpal joint is implicated the posteroanterior (PA)

glide of the proximal row of the carpal bones may be restricted. The testing of intercarpal gliding will specifically identify movement abnormalities between the proximal carpal bones and the adjacent radius or triangular fibrocartilage complex.

TREATMENT

Once the aggravating movement has been identified, an appropriate glide is chosen. The decision to use a weight-bearing or non-weight-bearing restricted movement will depend on the severity, irritability and nature of the condition (Maitland 1991). For example MWMs would preferably be

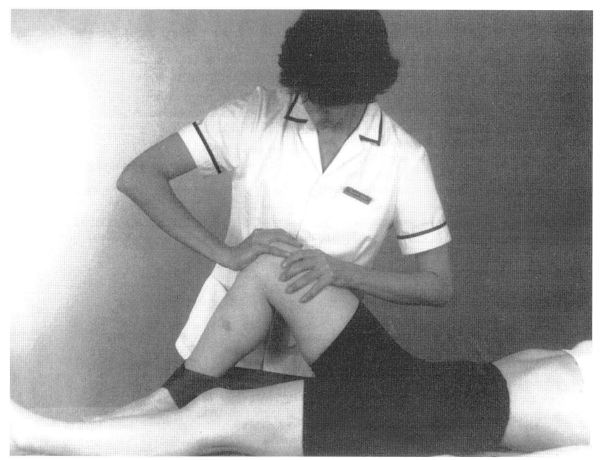

Figure 10.5 AP on the tibia with active flexion. (Reproduced with kind permission from *Physiotherapy* 1995 81(12): 726–729.)

performed in non-weight bearing if a patient with tibiofemoral limitation of extension had a history of recent trauma. Attempting to improve the same movement in weight bearing at this stage may further exacerbate the condition.

Once the glide has been chosen it must be sustained throughout the physiological movement until the joint returns to its original starting position. As the joint moves the therapist must sustain the pressure, being constantly aware of minor alterations in the treatment plane. The mobilizations performed are always into resistance but without pain. Immediate relief of pain and improvement in range of movement are expected. If this is not achieved the therapist may try a different glide or a rotation.

If pain-free movement is not achieved when performing an MWM a complex movement can be split into its various components and the MWM performed with one of the restricted single plane movements. For example, if a patient has tibiofemoral pain when performing a half squat, this movement involves a combination of flexion, adduction and medial rotation of the tibia. Medial rotation in flexion may be restricted and painful when tested in non-weight bearing. Performing an MWM at right angles or parallel to the joint line on active medial rotation in flexion in this non-weight-bearing position may achieve greater improvement in pain-free range than an MWM performed with the half squat. If pain relief is still not achieved then another manual treatment approach should be pursued. This clinical decision can be made instantly.

Clinical experience suggests that while sustaining the pain-free glide, the movement should be repeated 10 times. After this set of MWMs the joint function is re-assessed to see if the movement remains improved without the passive mobilization component. It may be necessary to repeat this set of 10 MWMs two to three times to ensure prolonged correction of tracking and sufficient afferent input. However, the number of repetitions is dependent on joint irritability. Taping can also be applied to help maintain joint position and increase proprioceptive awareness. Teaching the patient to perform their own MWMs is also useful to prolong pain-free move-

ment. Clinically, therapists using these techniques have often reported more instantaneous, dramatic results than those obtained when using repeated accessory or physiological passive mobilizations alone.

The following examples will illustrate the clinical application of MWMs to peripheral joints.

ANKLE INJURIES

The talocrural joint is relatively congruent and the gliding is usually successfully applied in the sagittal plane to improve plantar or dorsiflexion. The direction of the glide is determined using the concave/convex concept. An acute ankle sprain with limitation of dorsiflexion may be treated in non-weight bearing with the patient lying on the

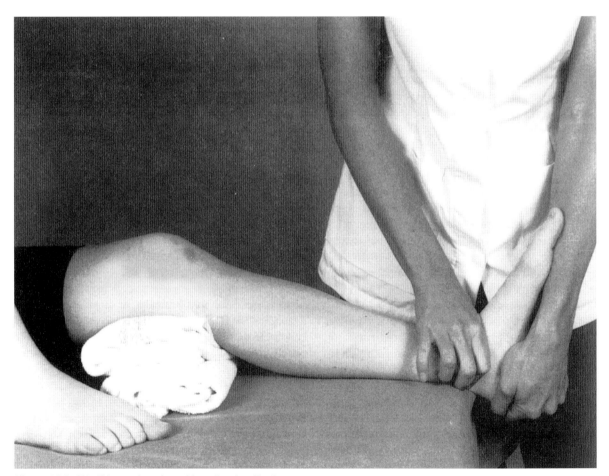

Figure 10.6 AP glide on the talus with active dorsiflexion.

treatment table with the ankle joint placed level with the end of the bed. A pillow placed under the knee will take the gastrocnemius off stretch. A sustained AP glide to the talus is applied by the therapist while the patient actively dorsiflexes the ankle. If the range of pain-free movement improves, the MWMs are repeated. Overpressure may be applied if pain-free end range is achieved (Fig. 10.6).

Mulligan (1995) has found that applying an AP/cephalad glide to the distal end of the fibula with active inversion often results in a dramatic improvement of inversion. This suggests that the dysfunction is more likely to be a joint surface problem rather than ligamentous in nature. In this case the talocrural or inferior tibiofibular joints are implicated. If the gliding of the talus relative to the mortise formed by the tibia and fibula does not result in pain-free inversion the inferior tibiofibular joint is implicated. There may be a history of previous inversion sprains and the patient may present to physiotherapy in the acute or chronic stage. Mulligan (1995) suggests that when the foot is inverted beyond the expected range the fibula is wrenched forward on the tibia with a positional fault occurring at the inferior tibiofibular joint. In that case the anterior talofibular ligament may remain virtually undamaged. Taping applied to the fibula whilst the therapist holds the AP glide can complement the treatment effects (Fig. 10.7).

In the post-acute stage of ankle sprain the residual functional disability may be an inability for the patient to lower himself downstairs on the injured ankle. MWMs can be performed with this movement by applying a PA glide on the tibia and fibula and a counter AP/cephalad glide on the talus applied with the therapist's web space, while the patient lowers himself down a step. The use of a belt to glide the tibia and fibula will help the therapist perform a stronger PA glide. If pain relief is not achieved with this, MWMs can be performed on the inferior tibiofibular joint an AP/PA direction (Fig. 10.8). The normal movement of the fibula with dorsiflexion is a cephalad glide and lateral rotation. This movement can be facilitated by angling the AP on the fibula correctly. It is important for the therapist to keep an

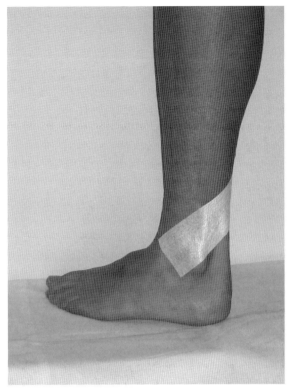

Figure 10.7 Corrective taping on fibula to maintain AP glide.

open mind: the direction of the MWM on the tibia and fibula is that which enables the patient to achieve pain-free movement.

NEURAL INVOLVEMENT IN SPRAINED ANKLES

Restoration of more normal articular biomechanics can permit greater mobility of the adjacent neural tissue (Butler 1991). This can also be applied in the periphery using MWM when adverse neurodynamics is a component of the restricted movement. By using MWMs the interface is moved actively relative to neural tissue in varying degrees of tension. The above techniques often improve signs and symptoms more rapidly than passive joint movement alone. The reasons for this are as yet unclear; theories hypothesizing why MWMs may have a normalizing effect on neurodynamics are discussed by Wilson (1994, 1995).

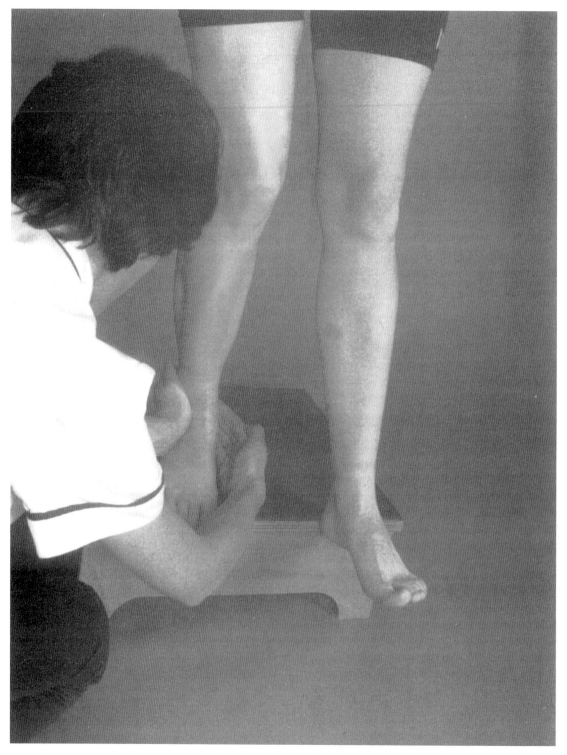

Figure 10.8 Gliding tibia and fibula with active end-range dorsiflexion. (Reproduced with kind permission from Physiotherapy 1995 81(12): 726–729.)

If, on assessment, inversion and plantarflexion are the symptomatic movements, and the symptoms are worsened by the addition of passive straight leg raise, the differential diagnosis indicates abnormal superficial peroneal nerve dynamics. Active inversion with a glide on the distal fibula in this same position of tension may result in the movement becoming symptom-free. The approach is to use the symptom-reducing glide as the treatment with the leg positioned in the same degree of straight leg raise. If a glide performed on the fibula in this position of tension can eliminate symptoms it is chosen as a treatment to be repeated with active inversion (Fig. 10.9). The head of the fibula is a bony interface of the common peroneal nerve and a potential tension site (Butler 1991). A glide on the head of the fibula may also be considered as a treatment option because the injury may have altered the position of the neck of the fibula relative to the common peroneal nerve. If there is no immediate change in symptoms it suggests that the nerve interface pathology may be soft tissue and more appropriate treatment must be given.

SHOULDER PATHOLOGY

The integrity of the shoulder complex is reliant largely on its ligamentous and muscular components (Hawkins et al 1991). Incorrect movement patterns can result in alterations of a joint's centre of rotation, which may cause cumulative microtrauma to the joint and its surrounding structures (Grant 1994). Common movement dysfunctions are frequently a result of incorrect scapula and rotator cuff musculature recruitment, a resulting downward-facing glenoid cavity and anterior or superior migration of the head of the humerus (Margery & Jones 1992; Jobe & Pink 1993).

Mobilizations with movements integrate well with muscle imbalance correction of these movement abnormalities. If the patient's problematic movement is abduction a corrective AP or longitudinal caudad glide on the head of the humerus can be sustained while the patient actively abducts the arm. The therapist's opposite hand fixates the scapula so that the

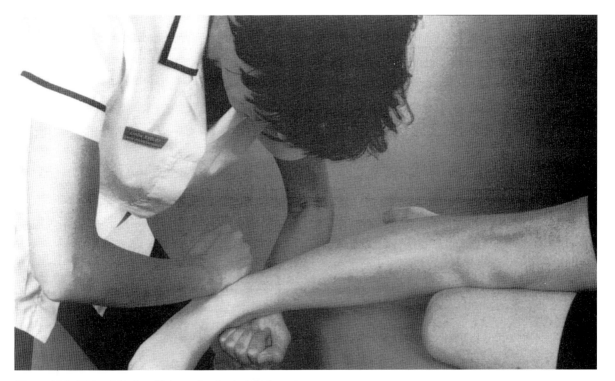

Figure 10.9 Glide of fibula with inversion in straight leg raise.

glide of the humerus is relative to the scapula. It is important to ensure that the AP glide is applied at right angles to the plane of the glenohumeral joint. The resulting movement must be pain-free. The patient can also be encouraged to activate specific muscles. For example, once a patient has been taught to activate a weak trapezius in isolation, the abduction MWM can be performed while encouraging correct recruitment of this muscle through the movement pattern (Fig. 10.10). Pain-free repetitions ensure sufficient corrective afferent input from the joint receptors and resulting reflex changes in muscle recruitment. A home programme of appropriate correct movement patterns (Sahrmann SA 2002) with the addition of taping will ensure prolonged and automatic pattern correction.

Similar glides can be applied if glenohumeral flexion is the symptomatic movement. A belt is usually used to glide the humeral head backward in the treatment plane, as the use of the ther-apist's hand over the anterior aspect of the head of the humerus will block the movement. A counter pressure is applied to the scapula from behind. It is essential that the belt is maintained at right angles to the plane of the joint. The belt position on the therapist should be lower than the glenohumeral joint; this ensures that the belt does not elevate the humeral head and impinge on superior structures. The belt and therapist position must be altered so that when the glide is applied the flexion is facilitated (Fig. 10.11).

CONCLUSION

The above clinical examples serve to illustrate the flexibility of this approach, which makes it highly suitable for integration into any therapist's favoured treatment regime, whatever their speciality.

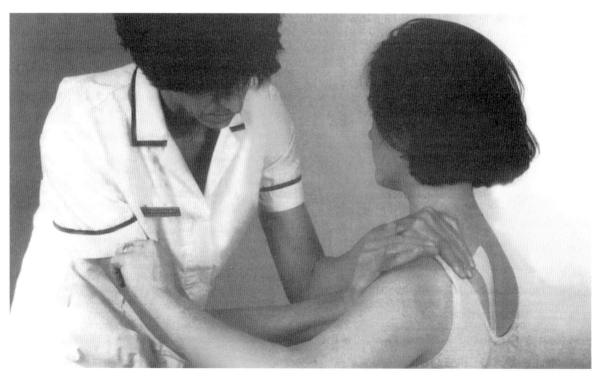

Figure 10.10 AP glide on humerus with active abduction and lower trapezius activation.

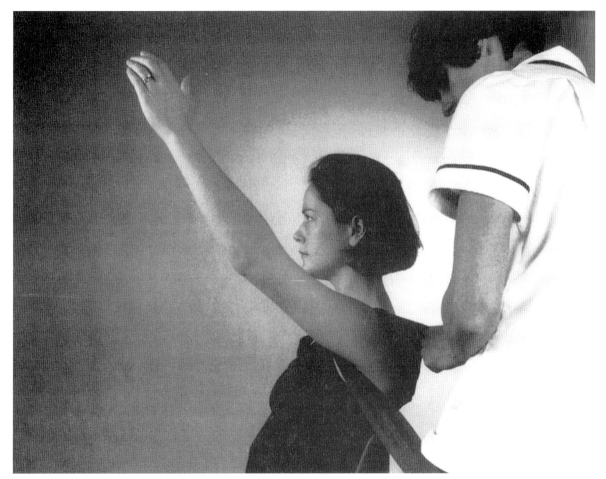

Figure 10.11 MWM with shoulder flexion.

Mobilization with movements enable the therapist to perform treatments in more dynamic, weight-bearing, functional positions. As the aggravating movement is used, treatment is specific and the results are often dramatic (Mulligan 1995). A single case study design by Vicenzino and Wright (1995) using this approach demonstrated improvement in a patient with tennis elbow. As this concept becomes established it is hoped that further research will be undertaken to substantiate the claims of 'immediate dramatic results'.

REFERENCES

Baxendale RH, Ferrell WR 1981 The effect of knee joint discharge on transmission in flexion pathways in decerebrate cats. Journal of Physiology 315: 231–242

Butler DS 1991 Mobilisation of the Nervous System Churchill Livingstone, Edinburgh, pp42, 185–210

Cobb CR, De Vries HE, Urban RT, Lcukens CA, Bugg RJ 1975 Electrical activity in muscle pain. American Journal of Physical Medicine 54: 80–87

Gerrard B, Matyas TA 1980 The electromyographic evaluation of an intervertebral mobilisation technique on cases presenting with acute paraspinal spasm in the lumbar spine. In: Proceedings of the Second Manipulative Therapists Association of Australia Conference, Adelaide pp 35–55

Grant R 1994 Physical Therapy of the Cervical and Thoracic Spine, 2nd edn. Churchill Livingstone, Edinburgh, p. 339

Hawkins RJ, Mohtadi GH 1991 Controversy in anterior shoulder instability. Clinical Orthopaedics and Related Research 272: 152–161

Jobe FW, Pink M 1993 Classification and treatment of shoulder dystunction in the overhead athlete. Journal of Orthopaedic and Sports Physical Therapy 18(2): 427–432

Kaltenborn FM 1989 Manual Mobilisation of the Extremity Joints, 4th edn. Orthopaedic Physical Therapy Products, USA, pp11, 20

Lewit K 1985 The muscular and articular factor in movement restriction. Manual Medicine 1: 83–85

Lundberg A, Malmgren K, Schonberg ED 1978 Role of the joint afferents in motor control exemplified by effects on reflex pathways from 1b afferents. Journal of Physiology 284: 327–343

Maitland GD 1991 Peripheral Manipulation, 2nd edn. Butterworths, London, p. 23

Margery M, Jones M 1992 Clinical diagnosis and management of minor shoulder instability. Australian Journal of Physiotherapy 38(4): 269–280

Mulligan BR 1993 Mobilisations with movement. Journal of Manual and Manipulative Therapy 1(4): 154–156

Mulligan BR 1995 Manual Therapy 'Nags', 'Snags', 'PRP's' etc., 3rd edn Plane View Services, Wellington, New Zealand

Murphy BA, Dawson NJ, Slack JR 1995 Sacroiliac joint manipulation decreases the H-reflex. Electromyography and Clinical Neurophysiology 35: 87–94

Sahrmann SA 2002 Diagnosis and Treatment of Movement Impairment Syndromes. Mosby, St Louis, USA

Schaible H, Grubb B 1993 Afferent and spinal mechanisms of joint pain. Pain 55: 5–54

Stokes M, Young A 1984 The contribution of reflex inhibition to arthrogenous muscle weakness. Clinical Science 67: 7–14

Taylor M, Suvinen T, Rheade P 1994 The effect of Grade 4 distraction mobilisation on patients with temporomandibular pain-dysfunction disorder. Physiotherapy Theory and Practice 10: 129–136

Thabe H 1986 EMG as a tool to document diagnostic findings and therapeutic results associated with somatic dysfunctions in the upper cervical spinal joints and sacroiliac joints. Manual Medicine 2: 53–58

Vicenzino B, Wright A 1995 Effects of a novel manipulative physiotherapy technique on tennis elbow: a single case study. Manual Therapy 1(1): 30–35

Williams P, (ed) 1995 Gray's Anatomy, 38th edn. Churchill Livingstone, Edinburgh, pp505–510

Wilson E 1994 Peripheral joint mobilisation with movement and its effects on adverse neural tension. Manipulative Physiotherapist 26(2): 35–40

Wilson E 1995 Mobilisation with movement and adverse neural tension: an exploration of possible links. Manipulative Physiotherapist 27(1): 40–46

POSTSCRIPT

A number of articles on peripheral MWM have been published since 1996. These encompass case reports (Backstrom 2002; Folk 2001), single case study designs (Vicenzino & Wright 1995; O'Brien & Vicenzino 1998), research investigating possible neurophysiological and mechanical effects (Kavanagh 1999; Vicenzino et al 2001; Abbott et al 2001a; Abbott et al 2001b; Hsieh et al 2002) and a randomized controlled trial (Kochar & Dogra 2002).

Using the Mulligan Concept a single case study design by Vicenzino and Wright (1995) demonstrated a long-term beneficial effect on a patient with tennis elbow. O' Brien and Vicenzino's study (1998) involved treating two patients with acute ankle sprains using a posterior glide to the distal end of the fibula with active ankle inversion. The results for both these subjects indicated that the MWM intervention produced an improvement in excess of that attributable to the natural history of a sprained ankle over a 5-week period.

Mulligan (1999) proposes that 'minor positional faults' may result in movement restriction. Folk's case study (2001) of a patient with a diagnosis that varied from a 'sprained' metacarpal joint of the thumb to De Quervain's tendinitis and finally to trigger thumb of the flexor sheath, seems to support this theory. Treatment included use of a splint, steroid injections into various tendon sheaths, surgical exploration and various electrotherapy modalities, but all these interventions were unsuccessful. The patient was finally referred to a manual therapist, who performed one treatment session of MWMs. This restored pain-free range of movement and function, which was maintained over a 1-year follow-up period.

The following two papers attempted to measure the positional fault. Using a potentiometer and strain gauge, Kavanagh (1999) measured AP excursion and force applied to the distal end of the fibula in 25 normal ankles and 6 acute sprained ankles. The sample size was too small to come to any definitive conclusions; however, nearly twice the AP force could be applied to the normal ankles compared with the ankle-sprain subjects. Pain was the limiting factor, however, thus questioning the ability to test a positional fault by measuring the amount of movement per unit of force. This method may be more applicable in less acute conditions. In the second paper Hsieh et al (2002) used magnetic resonance imaging (MRI) to measure the effect of MWM on thumb metacarpophalangeal (MCP) joint position. The pretreatment MRIs from the left and right MCP joints demonstrated a positional fault on the symptomatic side. An MRI taken while applying passive supination to the proximal phalanx demonstrated that the positional fault could be corrected. The patient was instructed to perform self MWMs for 3 weeks, which was reviewed on a weekly basis. The post-treatment MRI demonstrated that the positional fault was similar to that before treatment, even though the patient was pain-free and fully functional. This implies that the MWM produced its clinical effects through mechanisms more complex than long-term restoration of bony alignment.

Two papers that apply MWMs to a group of patients with tennis elbow may provide some clues to the neurophysiological responses (Abbott et al 2001a; Vicenzino et al 2001). The tennis elbow technique involves a sustained lateral glide to the elbow joint while contracting the extensor muscles of the forearm (Mulligan 1999). The results of these papers cannot be automatically extrapolated to the more traditional MWM, which involves applying a pain-free accessory glide to the *actively* moving joint. The sustained lateral elbow glide with gripping resulted in immediate significant changes in pain-free grip strength (Abbott et al 2001a). Vicenzino et al (2001) undertook a randomized, double-blind controlled study on tennis elbow patients and evaluated the effects of the same elbow lateral glide technique on pain-free grip strength (PFGS) and pressure pain threshold (PPT). This study demonstrated an immediate 50% increase in PFGS, with only a 10% increase in PPT. Of particular interest in these studies is that significant modulatory changes occurred in the motor neurone pool. However, the results of these papers only reflect *immediate* responses and are of limited clinical value when considered in isolation.

The clinical study by Kochar and Dogra (2002) provides some support to the laboratory findings. Their study randomized tennis elbow patients into two groups: one receiving ultrasound (US) and a graduated exercise programme and the other group receiving the elbow MWM technique and the same graduated exercise programme. A third group (control) received no treatment and did not attend the department on a regular basis. The treatment was administered for 10 sessions over 3 weeks. The graduated exercise regime was started after this 3-week period and continued for another 9 weeks. Outcome measures included pain assessed on a visual analogue scale, status of pain over the 24-hour period prior to assessment, grip strength and a 'weight test' that assessed the amount of weight the patient could lift free of pain with active wrist extension. At 3 weeks the MWM group were markedly better than the US group and control group in all parameters. After discharge, recovery continued over the 9 weeks

of exercise with the MWM group showing significantly greater improvement in all parameters. Pienimaki et al (1996, 1998) demonstrated the short- and long-term benefits of progressive strengthening and stretching exercises *only* when compared with ultrasound. Recent literature proposes that the majority of tendinopathies are more likely to be degenerative than inflammatory in nature and that an important component to their treatment is progressive strengthening incorporating eccentric loading (Khan et al 2000). The improvements in the objective tests of the MWM group may provide support to the proposal that there is a modulatory effect on the motor neurone pool, allowing faster progress with an exercise regime that may now be less inhibited by pain.

The greater part of the literature on this concept to date has been concerned with tennis elbow; hopefully the future will see more research on MWM intervention in other peripheral joints in order to establish the clinical efficacy of this valuable adjunct to manual therapy.

REFERENCES

Abbott JH, Patla CE, Jenson RH 2001a The initial effects of an elbow mobilisation with movement technique on grip strength in subjects with lateral epicondylalgia. Manual Therapy 6(3): 163–169

Abbott JH, Patla CE, Jenson RH 2001b Mobilisation with movement applied to the elbow affects shoulder range of motion in subjects with lateral epicondylalgia. Manual Therapy 6(3): 170–177

Backstrom KM 2002 Mobilisation with movement as an adjunct intervention in a patient with complicated De Quervain's tenosynovitis: A case report. Journal of Orthopaedic & Sports Therapy 32(3): 86–97

Folk B 2001 Traumatic thumb injury management using mobilization with movement. Manual Therapy 6(3): 178–182

Hsieh CY, Vicenzino B, Yang CH, Hu MH, Yang C 2002 Mulligan mobilisation with movement for the thumb: a single case report using magnetic resonance imaging to evaluate the positional fault hypothesis. Manual Therapy 7(1): 44–49

Kavanagh J 1999 Is there a positional fault at the inferior tibiofibular joint in patients with acute or chronic sprains compared to normals? Manual Therapy 4(1): 19–24

Khan KM, Cook JL, Maffulli N, Kannus P 2000 Where is the pain coming from in tendinopathy? It may be biochemical, not only structural, in origin. British Journal of Sports Medicine 34: 81–84

Kochar M, Dogra A 2002 Effectiveness of a specific physiotherapy regimen on patients with tennis elbow. Physiotherapy 88(6): 333–341

Mulligan BR 1999 Manual Therapy "Nags", "Snags", "MWMs" etc 4th edn Plane View Services, Wellington. New Zealand

O'Brien T, Vicenzino B 1998 A study of the effects of Mulligan's mobilisation with movement treatment of lateral ankle pain using a case study design. Manual Therapy 3(2): 78–84

Peinimaki T, Tarvainen TK, Sura PT, Vanharanta H 1996 Progressive strengthening and stretching exercises and ultrasound for chronic lateral epicondylitis. Physiotherapy 82(9): 522–530

Peinimaki T, Karinen P, Koivukangas P, Vanharanta H 1998 Long term follow-up of conservatively treated chronic tennis elbow patients: A prospective and retrospective analysis. Scandinavian Journal of Rehabilitation Medicine 30: 159–166

Vicenzino B, Paungmali A, Buratowski S, Wright A 2001 Specific manipulative therapy treatment for chronic lateral epicondylalgia produces uniquely characteristic hypoalgesia. Manual Therapy 6(4): 205–212

Vicenzino B, Wright A 1995 Effects of a novel manipulative physiotherapy technique on tennis elbow: a single case study. Manual Therapy 1(1): 30–35

Index